5 95 / PB

# THE SOFT FOODS
Cookbook

# THE SOFT FOODS Cookbook

Anne S. Chamberlain

Doubleday & Company, Inc.
Garden City, New York
1973

ISBN: 0-385-03284-6
Library of Congress Catalog Card Number 73-83587
Copyright © 1973 by Anne S. Chamberlain
All Rights Reserved
Published in the United States of America
First Edition

**FOR WARREN**

Whose courage will be remembered by all who knew and loved him

# CONTENTS

1. INTRODUCTION  1
   *Helpful Hints and General Information*

2. SEMI-SOFT MEALS  7

3. SEMI-SOFT AND BLENDED MEALS  39
   *Recipes that can be utilized for either type meals*

4. DESSERTS  89
   *Semi-soft and blended*

5. EXTRA NUTRITION  103
   *Suggestions and recipes for semi-soft and blended meals*

6. PREPARED FOODS 115
   *Source of supply—your supermarket*

7. FREEZING AND PLANNING AHEAD 119
   *Timesaving tips for busy days, visiting, and vacationing*

   INDEX 123

# THE SOFT FOODS
## Cookbook

## Chapter 1

# INTRODUCTION

## *Helpful Hints and General Information*

This book was written to meet the growing need of helping those people who have problems chewing or swallowing. The recipes range from semi-soft to blended meals, and are designed to solve the difficult problem of making the soft-food diet a tasty and nutritious one.

Most of the meals can be eaten by the whole family, thereby making the job of cooking easier for the person planning the menus. Also included are helpful hints for preparing quick and simple meals from prepared and frozen foods purchased at supermarkets. For those busy days these meals just require heating and, if necessary, blending.

By careful planning, the patient can still eat the same meals as the family, and, by blending and freezing, the person planning meals can have some days free of all the extra work of preparing soft-food menus.

My own experience covered four years of trying to devise meals for my own husband, who suffered from cancer. There were times he could eat food of a semi-soft nature, but many more when strictly blended foods only could be swallowed. The problem was to get beyond the bland dismaying fare of baby food and cooked cereals, which certainly are not adequate fare nutritionally for an adult, especially one who is ill and needs every ounce of energy-giving foods. I found nothing available that could help me, so by trial and error (literally!) I came up with the following recipes and helpful hints.

Chapter 2, Semi-soft Meals, is intended for those people who, for various reasons, have problems chewing or difficulty in swallowing anything rough. These meals need little or no chewing and are exceptionally moist, so there is no problem in swallowing.

The chapter for Semi-soft and Blended Meals can also be used for the family as well as anyone requiring a semi-soft diet; but these meals can readily be blended for those patients requiring a strictly liquefied diet. With these meals, even though in liquid form, they get a good nutritious meal, even including steak!

Equipment-wise, a blender, of course, is a necessity for a liquid diet. However, you can manage with a simple one—buying an expensive one with all kinds of buttons is not necessary. Mine had just two speeds and the "Off" button, and I managed very nicely with it.

An electric frying pan with a dome lid can be most helpful, but is not necessary—any frying pan or skillet would serve the same purpose for top-of-stove cooking—the important thing in most of the recipes is that it have a cover to help retain moisture.

Whenever browning any meat, be sure just to brown it

very lightly, turning frequently, as any coarse edges may be found irritating to the throat.

You can still serve a roast to the rest of the family, even though someone might be on a semi-soft or blended diet. Just be sure to have gravy (your own or canned). For a semi-soft diet, cut the meat into small pieces, adding a sufficient amount of gravy to make it good and moist, and serve with soft mashed potatoes and an easily swallowed vegetable. However, if blending is required, place gravy in blender first (this takes some of the load off the blender) and then add the cut-up meat. Potato and vegetable could be added with this mixture, or each served separately.

The same can be done for roast chicken or almost any type of roast, as long as you have the appropriate gravy to make it moist enough. Leftover roast or chicken can be used by cutting into bite-size pieces, mixed together with gravy, potato slices, either canned or uncooked, peas, and carrots, and simmered very slowly in a pan, covered. Simmer until vegetable and potato are cooked through, or just heat well if canned vegetables are used. This can be served as is for the family and a semi-soft diet, or a portion could be blended if required. Eggs are a good source of protein, and if one is on a semi-soft diet, a three-minute boiled egg will be no problem to eat. However, you can make an egg quite liquefied by boiling for only two minutes and adding a pat of butter, mixing well with a spoon before serving.

Canned soups are of tremendous help, and you will find a great variety containing meat, chicken, noodles, and vegetables providing good nourishment. For anyone on a semi-soft diet, most of them can be served according to directions on the can. However, if a liquefied diet is necessary, turn contents of the can into your blender, add half the can of milk or water—whatever is called for in that particular soup—and blend well. Then pour in the rest of the can and blend again. Be sure to follow these directions! The first time I thought of blending a can of soup, I emptied the entire can of milk into the blender after the contents of a can of cream of mushroom soup, pushed the "High" button on the blender, and swoosh—the whole top blew off and the kitchen cabinets and walls were well decorated with cream of mushroom soup! One of the "errors" of my "by trial and error." Speaking of soup, another of my "errors" was in trying to blend a can of oyster stew. Don't do it!—the taste is pretty bad.

A good lunch would be half of the soup mixture, a dish of ice cream, and a glass of milk. This could apply to a semi-soft diet as well as liquefied. If the person's appetite is poor, one of the heartier soups could be used as a main meal, supplemented with a milk shake or eggnog between meals for extra nutrition.

If the patient has little or no appetite, serve small portions made as attractive-looking as possible, perhaps at more frequent intervals if they will take it. Large amounts of food immediately tend to discourage one from eating. It is better to eat small amounts at more frequent intervals, if possible. If desired and permitted, alcoholic beverages can be an added source of nutrition. In fact, in some hospitals now, if a patient is on a liquid diet, he is permitted to keep beer or ale in the room or hospital refrigerator. It is considered a form of extra food, and, if he is used to having an occasional drink, gives him a little extra pleasure and relaxation, as well as extra nutrition. (In moderation of course!) Along this line, see Chapter 5, under Beverages, for the Eggnog recipe.

Chapter 7, Freezing and Planning Ahead, can be of much help for vacationing and visiting. This also I learned through trial and error—had a week's vacation, and at that time blended food was a necessity—but instead of spending much time "vacationing"—found myself blending and washing up after myself. The next week's vacation we had I didn't touch the blender once, and we were able really to enjoy ourselves.

Be sure you keep a good supply of canned soups and gravies on hand at all times—these will be very useful in preparing most of the recipes.

Last but not least, just because there is an eating problem in the family and you might not be able to go out to dinner to celebrate an extra-special occasion like a birthday or anniversary, you can still make a festive occasion of it at home.

Under Seafood in the Semi-soft and Semi-soft and Blended chapters, you will find a few extra-fancy meals, and in the Dessert chapter, a couple of special desserts to help keep the feeling of festivity and something special! The extra effort to make something special is well worth the trouble for the lift in spirits it gives to the patient as well as to the whole family. Use your best tablecloth and add candles, maybe a bit of champagne, and just see what it does for the morale!

## Chapter 2

# SEMI-SOFT MEALS

## General Information

These recipes can be eaten by the whole family as well as by anyone on a semi-soft diet—they require little or no chewing and are easily swallowed.

There are a variety of meals consisting of dairy products, meat, poultry, seafood, and vegetables. There are even a few open-faced sandwiches served with soups to make them moist enough to eat.

Some are in casserole form and others cooked in an electric frying pan or any pan, covered, for top-of-the-stove cooking. For baking or pan cooking, covering is very important, as it helps to retain moisture, thereby making it easier to chew and swallow.

Extra liquid, be it gravy or milk or whatever is called for in that particular recipe, can always be added if more moisture is required. You can decide according to what the patient needs.

## *Dairy Products*

### EGGS AND ASPARAGUS WITH CHEESE SAUCE

1 can (1 pound) asparagus
4 hard-cooked eggs, sliced
3 tablespoons butter or margarine
3 tablespoons flour
¾ teaspoon salt
Dash cayenne
2 cups milk
1 cup grated Cheddar cheese

Arrange asparagus on heatproof platter. Slice eggs and arrange on top of asparagus. In medium-size saucepan, blend melted butter or margarine, flour, salt, and cayenne. Gradually add milk. Stirring constantly, bring to boil over low heat and cook 1 minute, or until thick. Add the cheese and stir until melted. Pour contents of saucepan over asparagus and eggs in the heatproof platter. Broil approximately 6 inches from heat of broiler 3–5 minutes, or until top is bubbly and golden brown. Serves 4.

*Note:* This is a very nutritious meal for the whole family, and anyone on a semi-soft diet should find this very easy to eat.

# EGGS AND CORNED BEEF HASH

1 large can corned beef hash
4 eggs
Salt and pepper to taste

Open corned beef hash and divide into four equal slices. Place in frying pan and brown lightly on both sides.

Make an indentation with a spoon in the center of each slice after browning, and drop 1 egg on each slice.

Cover and simmer until egg is cooked. Season with salt and pepper. Serves 2–3.

*Note:* Be sure eggs are not overcooked; they should be in a soft and runny state to make the meal good and moist.

## EGGS ON RYE

6 slices bacon
2 tablespoons bacon drippings
½ cup chopped onion
⅓ cup chopped green pepper
8 eggs, slightly beaten
1 can cream of chicken soup
Dash pepper
1 tablespoon chopped pimiento
6 slices rye bread toasted or plain

In heavy skillet or frying pan, cook bacon until crisp; remove and crumble; set aside. In same pan, in bacon drippings, cook onion and green pepper until tender.

In separate bowl slightly beat the eggs, adding cream of chicken soup, pepper, pimiento, and bacon. Add this mixture to the onion and green pepper mixture, and cook over low heat until eggs are set; stir now and then. Serve on rye bread slices. Makes 6 open-faced sandwiches.

*Note:* About bacon bits—if the patient finds them difficult to swallow, remove enough of the mixture for his slice of bread, then add bacon bits to the mixture for the rest of the family and heat through.

## POACHED EGGS IN TOMATO SAUCE

2 tablespoons butter or margarine
1 large green pepper cut into thin strips
1 can (28 ounces) tomatoes
1½ teaspoons salt
⅛ teaspoon pepper
8 eggs

About 25 minutes before serving, in frying pan at medium-high heat melt butter or margarine, add green pepper, and cook about 5 minutes. Reduce to medium heat and add tomatoes, salt, and pepper. Cook 5 more minutes, or until pepper is tender.

Into simmering mixture, gradually and carefully drop eggs, one at a time. Cover and cook gently about 10 minutes, until eggs are just firm. Spoon vegetable mixture over eggs. Serves 4.

## "QUICK" CREAMED EGGS

1 can cream of mushroom soup
¼–½ cup milk
4 hard-cooked eggs, sliced
¼ cup chopped pimiento (optional)

Combine soup with milk in saucepan and heat thoroughly. Add eggs and pimiento, if desired. Stir gently. Serve hot and creamy on toast, plain bread, or soft open-faced buns. Serves 2–3.

## COTTAGE CHEESE PANCAKES

3 eggs, separated
1 cup small curd cottage cheese
¼ cup flour
2 tablespoons butter or margarine

Beat egg whites until stiff but not dry, and set aside. In separate mixing bowl beat yolks until light; add cottage cheese and flour, beating all together thoroughly. Lightly fold in egg whites.

Melt butter or margarine in skillet or frying pan, covering surface. Drop by tablespoons into size of pancakes desired and brown on both sides. Serves 3–4.

*Note:* These pancakes are exceptionally light and easy to swallow. By spreading butter or margarine on a pancake and adding maple syrup, anyone on a semi-soft diet should have no problem eating them.

## DEVILED MACARONI

1 cup elbow macaroni
3 tablespoons butter or margarine
2 tablespoons flour
1 teaspoon salt
1 teaspoon paprika
2 teaspoons prepared mustard
2 cups milk
½ cup grated Cheddar cheese
3 hard-cooked eggs
1 tablespoon French dressing
1 tablespoon milk
⅓ cup chili sauce
½ cup grated Cheddar cheese

Preheat oven to 375° F.

Cook elbow macaroni, drain, and set aside in 1½-quart baking dish. Melt butter or margarine in saucepan, stir in flour, salt, paprika, and mustard. Add 2 cups milk. Stir till thickened. Add ½ cup cheese. Pour over macaroni in baking dish.

Cut hard-cooked eggs in half. In separate dish mix yolks with French dressing and 1 tablespoon milk. Refill egg halves and place on top of casserole.

Mix chili sauce and ½ cup cheese and pour over egg halves in casserole. Bake about 20 minutes at 375° F. Serves about 6.

*Note:* This is a good recipe for anyone on a semi-soft diet and very nutritious. It could also be made in an electric frying pan, but be sure to keep cover on for extra moisture. Serve with salad or soft vegetable if patient cannot eat salad.

# *Meats*

## FRANKFURTERS ON RYE

6 frankfurters
⅓ cup chopped onion
2 tablespoons butter or margarine
6 slices rye bread, toasted or plain
6 large slices fresh tomato
1 can bean with bacon soup
⅓ can water
2 teaspoons prepared mustard
Pickle relish or pickles

Slash frankfurters diagonally at ½-inch intervals. In frying pan brown franks and onion in butter or margarine until done. Top each slice of bread with slice of tomato and 1 frankfurt.

Meanwhile, in saucepan, heat soup with water to rinse out can and mustard; stir now and then. Spoon sauce over sandwich. Garnish with relish or pickles if desired. Makes 6 open-faced sandwiches.

*Note:* The hot soup mixture softens the entire sandwich so it should be possible for anyone on a semi-soft diet to eat it. However, soft white bread or a soft white roll may be substituted.

## CREOLE HAMBURGER ON BUNS

1 pound hamburger
1 onion, chopped
1 green pepper, chopped
1 teaspoon salt
¼ teaspoon pepper
1 can (8 ounces) tomato sauce
½ cup water
½ cup corn flakes

In frying pan brown hamburger lightly. Add onion, green pepper, and season with salt and pepper. Add tomato sauce, rinsing out can with water. Add corn flakes and mix well. Simmer for about 15 minutes. Serve on sandwich or frankfurter rolls.

*Note:* This can be served to all the family as above directed. However, if a person is on a semi-soft diet, serve on open-faced rolls and add extra tomato sauce over the whole thing, making it extra moist; and he can eat with knife and fork instead of as a sandwich.

## HUNGARIAN GOULASH

2 cups elbow macaroni
1 tablespoon butter or margarine
1 tablespoon Parmesan grated cheese
1 pound ground beef
1 small onion, chopped fine
1 teaspoon parsley flakes
1 teaspoon celery flakes
1 teaspoon salt
½ teaspoon pepper
⅛ teaspoon chili powder
1 can (28 ounces) tomatoes

Cook elbow macaroni as directed on package, drain and put back into cooking pan. Stir in butter or margarine and cheese. Set aside. While elbows are cooking, brown beef lightly, together with onion, stirring frequently in frying pan. Add parsley flakes, celery flakes, salt, pepper, and chili powder, together with tomatoes. Mix thoroughly, and slowly add the cooked macaroni. Simmer, covered, stirring occasionally, about 30 minutes. Serves 6.

*Note:* This is very tasty and can be enjoyed by the whole family. Just be sure the hamburger is not too well browned and hard for the patient on a semi-soft diet. It is also an excellent one-dish meal.

## BACON-FLAVORED LIVER

2 slices bacon
1 pound beef liver
2 tablespoons flour
1 can tomato soup
½ can water
¼ cup chopped green pepper
¼ teaspoon chili powder

Cut bacon into small pieces and fry in pan until crisp; remove from pan. Dust liver in flour and brown lightly in bacon drippings, then remove any excess fat from pan.

Add tomato soup, using the water to rinse can, green pepper, and chili powder, stirring well. Cover and simmer on "Low" for 45 minutes, or until good and tender. Bacon bits may be added after liver is browned with the rest of the ingredients. Serves 2–3.

*Note:* If anyone has difficulty swallowing, the bacon bits might prove to be too sharp. Therefore, remove his portion of the meal before bacon bits are added for the rest of the family.

## SAUSAGE AND LIMA BEAN CASSEROLE

1 pound sausage, sweet or hot
1 onion, chopped fine
3 tablespoons sausage drippings
1 can tomato soup
2 packages frozen baby lima beans
½ can lima bean stock
½ teaspoon salt
Pinch poultry seasoning

In frying pan, brown sausage lightly, together with onion. Sausage may be left whole, but it is preferable that it be cut into 1-inch-long pieces. Remove excess fat except for 3 tablespoons. Add tomato soup.

Meanwhile, while sausage is browning, cook lima beans according to directions on package, drain, reserving bean stock to rinse out can of tomato soup. Add this stock to sausage and soup mixture, together with salt and poultry seasoning. Pour drained lima beans into frying pan, stirring well. Simmer slowly, covered, about 45–50 minutes, or until sausage is tender. Serves 4–5.

*Note:* The above can be poured into a 1½-quart baking dish and baked at 350° F. for about 1 hour if preferred, with a cover for extra moisture. Also, more bean stock or soup can be added if additional moisture is desired.

## ECONOMICAL VEAL PARMESAN

1 package breaded veal steaks
1 tablespoon salad oil
1 small onion, chopped fine
2 cans (8 ounces each) tomato sauce
1 small mozzarella cheese (about 6 ounces)

Brown veal steaks in oil, together with chopped onion, very lightly, in frying pan. Pour tomato sauce over all, and simmer very slowly on "Low," approximately 45 minutes. Slice mozzarella cheese, placing slices on top of veal steaks, and continue to simmer until cheese is melted. Spoon sauce over each steak occasionally while simmering. Serves 4.

*Note:* The packaged breaded veal steaks are very soft, and with sufficient sauce and cut into small pieces, almost anyone on a semi-soft diet should be able to eat them.

## SAVORY VEAL STEAK

1 pound veal steaks, cut thin
2 tablespoons flour
2 tablespoons salad oil
2 small onions, sliced thin
½ teaspoon salt
½ teaspoon pepper
¼ teaspoon paprika
½ cup light sour cream

Cut veal steaks into serving-size pieces, roll in flour, and brown lightly in salad oil in frying pan or heavy skillet, together with onions. Sprinkle with salt, pepper, and paprika, then place onions on top of veal steaks. Add sour cream, cover, and simmer over low heat about 1 hour, or until steak is tender. If mixture should start to become a bit dry, add more milk to keep good and moist.

*Note:* The whole family can enjoy this, and for anyone requiring soft food, just be sure to cut the meat into very small pieces, adding plenty of the liquid.

## VEAL AND EGG TERRAPIN

2 hard-cooked eggs
1 cup leftover roast veal, cut in bite-size pieces
3 tablespoons butter or margarine
1 onion, minced
¾ teaspoon salt
¼ teaspoon pepper
¼ teaspoon marjoram
3 tablespoons flour
1½ cups milk
¼ teaspoon bottled meat sauce
Chopped parsley (optional)

Remove shells from eggs and cut into wedges. Set eggs and veal aside. Melt butter or margarine in saucepan, add onion, together with salt, pepper, and marjoram. Cook until onion is clear.

Remove from heat, stir in flour and gradually add milk. Return to medium heat, cook and stir until thickened and smooth, about 5 minutes. Add meat sauce, pieces of veal, and eggs.

Heat thoroughly and serve on soft rolls, toast, or cooked noodles. Garnish with sprinkling of chopped parsley if desired. Serves 2–3.

*Note:* For the person on a semi-soft diet, according to his condition or ability this could be served as is, on soft white bread, or on very soft mashed potatoes.

## VEAL PARMESAN

1 egg, beaten
½ teaspoon salt
¼ teaspoon pepper
1 cup flour or bread crumbs
1 pound veal steaks, cut very thin
1 tablespoon salad oil
1 small onion, chopped fine
2 small cans (8 ounces each) tomato sauce
1 small mozzarella cheese (about 6 ounces)

In a bowl, place the egg, beaten together with salt and pepper, and in another bowl put the flour or bread crumbs. Dip each veal steak first into the egg mixture and then in the flour or bread crumbs. Heat salad oil in frying pan, add onion, and brown veal steaks lightly. Pour tomato sauce over all, and cook very slowly on low simmer approximately 45 minutes. Slice mozzarella cheese, and place a slice on top of each veal steak, continuing to simmer until cheese is melted. Spoon tomato sauce over each occasionally while simmering. Keep covered, as this helps to maintain moisture. Serves 4–5.

*Note:* This is especially tasty and can easily be eaten by someone on a semi-soft diet. Just be sure to keep it good and moist with enough tomato sauce, and cut it into very small pieces with ample sauce, so he can chew and swallow with little or no effort.

# *Poultry*

## CHICKEN AND ELBOWS CASSEROLE

1½ cups elbow macaroni
1 can cream of mushroom soup
½–¾ can milk
1 teaspoon parsley flakes
1 teaspoon celery flakes
Dash chili powder
Salt and pepper to taste
1 can (6½–7 ounces) chicken
Grated Cheddar cheese (optional)

Cook elbow macaroni as directed on package, drain, and place in covered frying pan. In saucepan, place contents of cream of mushroom soup, using milk to rinse out can; add parsley and celery flakes and chili powder, with salt and pepper to taste. Mix well. Turn out contents of can of chicken, drained and flaked. Stir all together until well heated and thoroughly blended. Add contents of saucepan to elbow macaroni, stir well, and cover. Simmer until well heated, stirring occasionally. Serves 6.

*Note:* This can also be baked by placing elbow macaroni in a 1½-quart casserole dish and adding the contents of the saucepan. Optional: Sprinkle grated Cheddar cheese over top of casserole. Keep covered for additional moisture. Bake approximately 30 minutes at 350° F.

# *Seafood*

Fish is a source of good nutrition, and the recipes following should meet the taste of almost everyone.

## TUNA AND ELBOW MACARONI CASSEROLE

1½ cups elbow macaroni
1 can cream of mushroom soup
½–¾ cup milk
Salt and pepper to taste
1 teaspoon parsley flakes
1 teaspoon celery flakes
Dash chili powder
1 can (6½–7 ounces) tuna fish
Grated Cheddar cheese (optional)

Cook elbow macaroni as directed on package, drain, and place in frying pan with cover. In saucepan, turn out contents of cream of mushroom soup can, using milk to rinse out can. Add salt and pepper, parsley and celery flakes, chili powder, and tuna fish, drained and flaked. Stir until thoroughly mixed. Add contents of saucepan to the elbow macaroni and mix well. Cover and simmer slowly until heated through; stir occasionally. Serves 4–5.

*Note:* If desired, the above recipe can be poured into a 1½-quart casserole, sprinkled with a little Cheddar cheese, then baked in 350° F. oven for 30 minutes. Be sure to keep covered to retain moisture.

## FILLETS 'N SHRIMP

1 pound fillets (haddock or any you prefer)
8 soda biscuits
1 can cream of shrimp soup
½ cup milk

Preheat oven to 350° F.

Place fillets on an oiled baking dish. Crush soda biscuits and sprinkle on top of fillets, covering well. Open can of cream of shrimp soup and place in bowl, adding milk, and mix thoroughly. Pour on top of crushed biscuits. Bake in 350° F. oven approximately 45 minutes. Serves 4.

*Note:* A heavy skillet or an electric frying pan could also be used for this recipe. However, if it has a Teflon finish, very little oil will be needed. Just add ingredients as above, cover, and simmer approximately 45 minutes.

If the family likes seafood, this is very tasty, and so soft that anyone requiring soft food would have no difficulty eating it.

## LOBSTER NEWBURG

¼ pound butter or margarine
1 tablespoon flour
1 pint cream
2 jiggers cooking sherry
1 can frozen lobster meat, or 1 pound fresh, if available

In saucepan, blend butter or margarine with flour, mixing thoroughly. Add cream, cooking slowly and stirring until slightly thickened. Add cooking sherry and drained lobster meat, simmering slowly until heated through. Serve over lightly toasted bread. Serves 2–3.

*Note:* Lobster meat does not as a rule blend very well, but can be used readily for a semi-soft diet, as it requires little or no chewing.

This is a good meal for that festive occasion!

## TOMATO CURRY LOBSTER TAILS

6 frozen rock lobster tails, about 10 ounces each
2 tablespoons butter or margarine
½ cup minced onion
1 garlic clove
½ cup chopped green pepper
1 can (16 ounces) tomatoes
2 teaspoons curry powder
1 teaspoon salt
1 bay leaf

Boil lobster tails as directed on package. Cut away underside membrane and remove meat from shells; cut meat into bite-size pieces and reserve empty shells.

In large saucepan over medium heat, melt margarine or butter. Add minced onion, garlic, and green pepper, and cook until tender but not brown. Add tomatoes, curry powder, salt, and bay leaf. Cover and cook over low heat 10 minutes, stirring occasionally. Add cut-up lobster meat and simmer until heated through, about 5 minutes. Remove garlic and bay leaf. Fill reserved lobster shells with mixture and serve hot. Serves 6.

*Note:* This is another meal which can be used for that special occasion and still easily eaten by anyone on a semi-soft diet.

## OYSTER-TUNA CASSEROLE

1½ cups elbow macaroni
2 tablespoons butter or margarine
1½ tablespoons flour
1 can oyster stew
1 cup diced processed Cheddar cheese
1 can (6½–7 ounces) tuna fish
Thin tomato wedges (optional)

Preheat oven to 375° F.

Cook elbow macaroni as directed on package. While elbows are cooking, melt butter or margarine in large saucepan, stir in flour and liquid drained from oyster stew. Cook, stirring until smooth. Add cheese, simmering slowly until cheese is melted. Drain elbows when done and add to mixture in saucepan, stirring well. Add tuna fish, drained and flaked, and oysters from can of oyster stew which have been set aside. Mix thoroughly and pour into shallow 1½-quart baking dish, dot top with thin tomato wedges if desired, and bake at 375° F. for 15–20 minutes. Serves 4–5.

*Note:* Do *not* blend this recipe, as oysters do not blend well.

This can be eaten by the whole family, and for anyone on a semi-soft diet, be sure and keep covered to retain moisture.

## *Vegetables*

Vegetables are an important part of anyone's diet, and the patient should be encouraged to eat them whenever possible. According to season, vegetables are on the whole plentiful, and can be utilized according to the patient's ability to chew or swallow and, of course, his own personal likes and dislikes.

Carrots are especially nutritious and available year round and can readily be used for a semi-soft diet by adding sufficient butter or margarine. If blending is necessary, add extra butter or margarine and milk to obtain the desired consistency. Cauliflower is another vegetable that blends well with the addition of butter or margarine and milk and is nice and creamy. In fact, almost any of the fresh vegetables could be blended—just add extra milk or butter, or some of that good nutritious liquid they are cooked in, which is usually drained down the sink! To further make use of these vegetables, you will find a few recipes next that can be made into entire meals.

## EGGPLANT PARMESAN

1 large eggplant
1 cup flour
2 eggs
3 tablespoons milk
½ teaspoon salt
¼ teaspoon pepper
2 tablespoons salad oil
Grated Parmesan cheese
1 jar (15½ ounces) tomato sauce (plain or with
   meat) or your own tomato sauce and meatballs

Preheat oven to 350° F.
Remove skin from eggplant and slice in medium-thin slices. Using two separate bowls, place flour in one, and eggs, milk, salt, and pepper in the other, and beat well with fork. Dip each slice of eggplant first in flour and then in milk and egg mixture, and brown lightly in salad oil in frying pan. More oil may have to be added as you continue frying slices, depending on the size of the eggplant.
In casserole dish, cover bottom lightly with tomato sauce, place a layer of eggplant, spoon more sauce over slices, then sprinkle grated cheese. Continue alternating layers, finishing with a topping of sauce to cover completely the top layer, adding meatballs if desired. Sprinkle more

cheese for topping. Bake at 350° F. about 40–50 minutes. Serves 6.

*Note:* If you use enough sauce to retain moisture well, this is a good recipe for a semi-soft diet. Just be sure to keep dish covered while baking.

## MUSHROOM PIE

2 tablespoons butter or margarine
¼ cup diced onion
2 cups hot cooked, sieved potatoes
1 can (3 ounces) chopped broiled mushrooms
1 pound creamed cottage cheese
½ cup sour cream
1 teaspoon salt
⅛ teaspoon pepper
½ teaspoon Gravymaster
2 eggs, well beaten
1 9-inch pastry shell, unbaked

Preheat oven to 375° F.
Melt butter or margarine in small saucepan, add onion, and cook over moderate heat 5 minutes, stirring occasionally. Into potatoes stir mushrooms, cottage cheese, sour cream, salt, pepper, Gravymaster, and cooked onions from small saucepan. Mix thoroughly. Fold in eggs, well beaten, and pour into pastry shell. Bake at 375° F. about 1 hour, or until puffy and lightly brown. Serve hot as main dish. Serves 4.

*Note:* For anyone with swallowing problems who finds the pastry shell too difficult to swallow, just remove shell from his portion.

## BAKED STUFFED PEPPERS WITH BEEF RAVIOLI

4 medium-size green peppers
1 can (14½ ounces) tomato sauce
1 can (15½ ounces) beef ravioli
¼ cup grated Parmesan cheese

Preheat oven to 350° F.

Wash peppers, cut in half lengthwise, removing seeds and membranes. Boil for approximately 5 minutes, until softened a bit, then drain. Pour contents of can of tomato sauce into greased shallow baking dish; then place pepper halves cut side up in sauce. Fill each pepper half with beef ravioli. Top with Parmesan cheese. Bake at 350° F. for 30–40 minutes. Serves 3–4.

*Note:* For extra moistness, be sure to keep dish covered while baking for anyone on a semi-soft diet.

## BAKED STUFFED PEPPERS WITH CORNED BEEF HASH

4 medium-size green peppers
1 can (15 ounces) corned beef hash
1 egg
1 small onion, chopped fine
1 teaspoon parsley flakes
1 teaspoon celery flakes
Dash chili powder
½ teaspoon salt
¼ teaspoon pepper
1 can (14½ ounces) tomato sauce

Preheat oven to 350° F.

Wash and clean out inside of green peppers, removing seeds and membrane, leaving pepper intact except for hole in top. Simmer in small amount of water in covered saucepan until tender but easy to handle; drain. In mixing bowl empty contents of can of corned beef hash, add egg, onion, parsley and celery flakes, chili powder, salt and pepper; mix well. When peppers are cool enough to handle, stuff with hash mixture from mixing bowl and place in baking dish. Pour tomato sauce over stuffed peppers, cover baking dish, and bake at 350° F. for 30–40 minutes. Serves 4.

*Note:* This is another meal for the family as well as for one on a soft diet, as the corned beef hash has potatoes in it; so you get meat, vegetables, and potato in one dish.

## BAKED STUFFED TOMATOES WITH CELERY CREAM SAUCE

2 tablespoons butter or margarine
1 teaspoon finely chopped onion
2½ cups soft bread cubes
½ teaspoon salt
¼ teaspoon pepper
6 firm ripe tomatoes
1 can (10½ ounces) condensed cream of celery soup
½ cup milk

Preheat oven to 375° F.

Melt butter or margarine and cook onion until soft. Combine soft bread cubes, salt, pepper, and mix well. Wash tomatoes, remove stem end, and scoop out pulp; cut up pulp and add to bread mixture. Stuff tomato shells with mixture and place in greased baking dish. Turn out contents of the can of cream of celery soup, adding ½ cup milk to rinse out can; simmer about 2 minutes. Pour over stuffed tomatoes, cover baking dish, and bake at 375° F. about 20 minutes. Makes approximately 6 servings.

*Note:* If the bits of celery should be difficult to swallow, the soup mixture could be blended first before pouring over tomatoes.

## Chapter 3

# SEMI-SOFT AND BLENDED MEALS

## General Information

The recipes in this chapter consist again of meals that may be served to the whole family, as well as for a semi-soft diet—but best of all, they can readily be used for a blended diet. The food may be made more or less liquefied by the amount of whatever liquid is called for in that particular recipe. For instance, the more milk that is added, the more readily it may be poured even into a glass or cup.

You could make good use of a thermos bottle for really liquefied meals should you desire to make a day trip or go visiting. It is kept good and hot and requires no heating—another convenience. Personally, I've even prepared some of these meals and taken them to the hospital in a thermos, when hospital fare proved to be inedible at the time.

Anyone on a strictly liquid diet, for whatever reason, does not have to settle for just broths or milk shakes, etc. They can even have steak and all the nourishment of a complete meal!

Before we go on with the recipes, this bears repeating: Keep a good variety of soups and gravies on hand. These are a must for a blended diet, as well as being most helpful in a semi-soft diet.

# *Meats*

## BEEF STEW

1 pound beef stew meat
1 cup flour
1 teaspoon salt
½ teaspoon pepper
2 tablespoons salad oil
1 small onion, chopped fine
1 teaspoon parsley flakes
1 teaspoon celery flakes
1 teaspoon garlic salt
2 tablespoons Gravymaster
¼ teaspoon chili powder
¼ teaspoon crushed red pepper
3 medium onions
1 bunch carrots
2 medium potatoes
8–10 cups water

Cut stew meat into very small cubes, about ½-inch square. This is done more easily when meat is slightly frozen. Place flour together with salt and pepper into a paper bag, add the cut-up meat, and shake well until meat is thoroughly coated with flour. In large skillet warm salad oil, add 1 small onion, chopped fine, and cook until partially soft; add meat and brown lightly. When meat is browned on all sides, add parsley flakes, celery flakes, garlic salt, Gravymaster, chili powder, crushed red pepper, and enough water, about 2 cups, to cover entire mixture and mix well. Simmer on lowest heat for about 1 hour, stirring occasionally, and adding water if necessary to keep from sticking. Add 3 medium onions, cut into wedges, and 2–3 cups more of water and continue simmering for another hour. Meanwhile, peel and cut into very small cubes the carrots and potatoes and add to contents of skillet, along with 5 or 6 more cups of water. Stir well, and after this has simmered for a while, about another hour, taste it and add more condiments or water according to your own taste and the consistency you desire. Cooking time should be no less than 4 hours, simmering slowly, to make a really good, tender, tasty stew.

*Note:* The reason for cutting the meat and vegetables into such small cubes is that it makes it possible for one on a semi-soft diet to swallow it more readily. If blending is desired, it makes less of a strain on the blender to add gravy first, and makes a very nutritious and tasty meal. The more gravy you add, the more liquefied the results.

## CHUCK ROAST—SKILLET STYLE

1 tablespoon salad oil
3-pound boned chuck roast
1 teaspoon salt
½ teaspoon pepper
½ teaspoon garlic salt
1 can cream of mushroom soup
4 medium-size potatoes
1 bunch carrots

In frying pan or heavy skillet heat the salad oil. Add chuck roast, sprinkling with salt, pepper, and garlic salt, and brown lightly on both sides. Drain off any excess oil after browning. Open can of cream of mushroom soup and turn entire contents over top of roast, letting excess fall over sides into the frying pan. Turn to low simmer and cook for about 1½ hours. Meanwhile, pare potatoes and carrots, cutting potatoes into quarters and carrots into fairly thin slices; place around the roast and continue to simmer gently. After ½ hour, take top off frying pan and baste potatoes and carrots with juices that have accumulated. Do this every ½ hour or so until just tender. Cooking time might vary according to the size of the roast, but usually about 3 hours will be sufficient. Serves 4–5.

*Note:* This makes an exceptionally moist and tender piece of meat, besides being inexpensive and something the whole family can eat. If the cut of meat you get is not too good, just simmer a little longer until it is tender. Cut into small pieces and served with gravy, it should pose no problem to one on a semi-soft diet. This can also be blended by adding gravy to the blender first, then the meat and vegetables. If more moisture is required, add ½ can milk to the soup mixture. This makes a well-balanced meal, hearty and nutritious for anyone requiring a liquefied diet.

## MEAT LOAF

1 pound ground beef
2 eggs, slightly beaten
¼ cup chopped onion
2 teaspoons salt
¼ teaspoon pepper
1 teaspoon celery flakes
1 teaspoon parsley flakes
Dash chili powder
2 teaspoons grated Parmesan cheese
1 cup rolled oats (quick cooking) or soft bread crumbs
1 can beef or mushroom gravy

Preheat oven to 350° F.

In large bowl mix together the following: ground beef, eggs, chopped onion, salt, pepper, celery and parsley flakes, chili powder, and Parmesan cheese.

After this has been mixed thoroughly, add rolled oats (or soft bread crumbs) plus half the can of beef or mushroom gravy. Pat combined mixture into greased loaf pan, pouring remaining half of gravy over meat. Bake in 350° F. oven approximately 1 hour. Serves 4–5.

*Note:* By adding sufficient gravy over a slice of meat loaf, this can be used on a semi-soft diet, together with mashed potatoes and soft vegetable. However, if blending is needed, add gravy to blender and then place broken meat loaf slice into the blender, until of proper consistency for individual. Add a blended vegetable and potato for a well-balanced meal.

## MEAT LOAF WITH MUSHROOM STUFFING

1 can (3 ounces) sliced mushrooms
¼ cup minced onion
⅛ cup butter or margarine
2 cups fresh soft bread crumbs
⅛ teaspoon powdered thyme
⅛ cup minced parsley
1 pound ground beef
1 egg, slightly beaten
¾ teaspoon salt
¼ teaspoon pepper
¼ cup catsup
¼ cup mushroom broth

Preheat oven to 350° F.

Drain the mushrooms, reserving broth, and sauté with onion in butter or margarine until onion is transparent. Combine with bread crumbs, thyme, and parsley. In separate bowl, lightly mix together the ground beef, egg, salt, pepper, catsup, and mushroom broth. Place half of meat mixture in loaf pan, making a smooth layer, pack mushroom stuffing on top, and then add remainder of meat mixture. Bake in 350° F. oven for approximately 40–45 minutes. Drain excess juices if desired. Serves 4–5.

*Note:* This should be soft and moist enough for anyone on a semi-soft diet; however, if more moisture is necessary, open and heat a can of mushroom gravy to ladle over the patient's serving. For blending, pour ½ can of mushroom gravy into blender first, and then a slice of meat loaf, broken into small pieces. By adding blended potato and vegetable, this also makes a well-balanced meal.

## MEAT-ZA-PIE

1 pound ground beef
½ teaspoon salt
½ cup bread crumbs
⅔ cup evaporated milk
½ cup tomato sauce
2–3 slices American processed cheese
¼ teaspoon orégano
Grated Parmesan cheese

Preheat oven to 350° F.
Place ground beef, salt, and bread crumbs in 9-inch pie plate. Add evaporated milk and mix well with fork. Spread mixture evenly over bottom of pan, preferably using the heel of your hand for best results, and raising a rim about ½ inch high around the side of the pie plate. Spread tomato sauce over meat mixture. Cut 2–3 slices of American cheese into strips and arrange in crisscross pattern over top. Sprinkle with orégano and Parmesan cheese, giving the meat a light dusting. Bake in 350° F. oven about 30 minutes or until cheese is melted and meat is cooked through. Serves 4–5.

*Note:* This is good for the whole family as well as for one on a semi-soft diet; just be sure it is not overcooked to the point where the edges of meat are overdone and sharp. By adding a little extra tomato sauce to the blender before the meat, it can also be used on a blended diet. The amount of sauce used would depend on the consistency desired. Depending on the patient's appetite, a blended vegetable could be added.

## OVEN BEEF ROAST

Large piece of aluminum foil—big enough to wrap entire roast and fold over
4–5 pound top round roast
Salt and pepper to taste
1 can cream of mushroom soup
¼–½ envelope of onion soup mix

Preheat oven to 450° F.

Place large sheet of aluminum foil in roasting pan and arrange top round roast in center. Sprinkle with salt and pepper to taste. Turn out contents of can of cream of mushroom soup on top of roast, letting excess slide around it. Sprinkle onion soup mix over all. Fold aluminum foil across the top and on either side, lifting center of fold gently upwards so it doesn't press down on meat. Bake in hot oven at 450° F., approximately 20–25 minutes per pound. At the end of 1½ hours, remove from oven and test for rareness according to liking. If it is done through enough for your taste, fold aluminum foil back and return to oven for 10–15 minutes more, to brown lightly on top. Remove meat to cutting board and pour juices into small saucepan to make gravy, or use the juices as is if you prefer. Serves 6.

*Note:* Baking a roast in this manner makes it exceptionally tender. A chuck roast could also be used if a less expensive cut is desired. However, if it is to be used for a semi-soft diet, the better cut is preferable. Cut into very small pieces, pouring gravy over the meat. If blending is required, add gravy to the blender first and then the cut-up meat. A chuck roast could easily be used for this purpose.

## RICE AND BEEF PORCUPINES

1 pound ground beef
½ cup Minute Rice
3 tablespoons chopped onion
1 teaspoon salt
¼ teaspoon pepper
¼ teaspoon poultry seasoning
3 tablespoons salad oil
2 cans (8 ounces each) tomato sauce
1 cup water

In large bowl mix well together, the ground beef, Minute Rice, chopped onion, salt, pepper, and poultry seasoning. Form into small balls and brown lightly in salad oil in frying pan or heavy skillet. Drain off excess oil. Add tomato sauce and water, cover, and simmer slowly about 50 minutes. Serves 4–5.

*Note:* Served with a favorite vegetable, this makes a well-balanced meal and can be eaten as is for a semi-soft diet. If blending is necessary, place tomato sauce in blender first and then add whatever number of meat balls the patient might desire. Add a blended vegetable if his appetite is good. If not, keep the beef portion to a reasonable amount so as to get a more balanced meal by including a blended vegetable.

## SKILLET ZUCCHINI AND BEEF

1 medium onion, chopped fine
1 medium green pepper, chopped fine
1 tablespoon salad oil
1 pound ground beef
1 can (16 ounces) stewed tomatoes
1 can (6 ounces) tomato paste
1 teaspoon salt
½ teaspoon orégano
¼ teaspoon garlic powder
2 medium zucchini, cut into ¼-inch slices

In frying pan over medium heat, cook onion and green pepper in salad oil until tender. Add ground beef and stir until lightly brown. Add stewed tomatoes, tomato paste, salt, orégano, and garlic powder; stir and simmer about 10 minutes. Add zucchini and cook covered 10–15 minutes, until zucchini is tender. Makes approximately 5–6 servings.

*Note:* This makes an excellent meal for the whole family and for anyone on a semi-soft diet, as long as you are careful not to get the ground beef too crisp. It may also be blended for someone on a liquefied diet. Just before serving the rest of the family, place enough in the blender for 1 serving and let blend while getting the rest of the meal on the table. Extra portions could also be blended for the freezer for a future quick meal or for vacationing or visiting.

## TOMATO MEAT BALLS WITH NOODLES

1 pound ground beef
1 small onion, chopped
1 teaspoon salt
¼ teaspoon thyme
½ cup dry bread crumbs
1 egg, slightly beaten
1 can tomato soup
⅓ cup water
1 tablespoon butter or margarine
1 package (6 ounces) noodles, cooked

Mix ground beef, onion, salt, thyme, bread crumbs, and egg together; form into 6 large or 12 small meat balls. In saucepan combine tomato soup and water to rinse out can, and heat to boiling point. Drop meat balls into soup mixture, cover, and let simmer about 50 minutes. Add butter or margarine to cooked noodles, stirring until butter is absorbed; place on serving platter. Pour soup and meat ball mixture over noodles. Makes approximately 6 servings.

*Note:* This is another meal the whole family can enjoy, as well as anyone on a semi-soft diet. The meat balls and soup mixture could be blended and served with a blended vegetable, making a well-balanced meal.

## TOP OF STOVE MEAT LOAF

1 pound ground beef
½ cup dry bread crumbs
1 can tomato soup
¼ cup finely chopped onion
1 egg, slightly beaten
1 teaspoon salt
¼ teaspoon pepper
1 tablespoon shortening
½ cup water
½ teaspoon prepared mustard
2 slices processed cheese, cut in half

In large bowl, mix the following thoroughly: ground beef, bread crumbs, ¼ cup of tomato soup, chopped onion, 1 egg, salt, and pepper. Shape firmly into two loaves; brown lightly in shortening in frying pan or heavy skillet. Cover and cook over low heat for 25 minutes. Spoon off excess fat. Pour remaining soup mixed with water and prepared mustard over loaves, and top with cheese slices. Cook about 10 minutes uncovered, until cheese is melting and warm. Baste with soup mixture during this 10 minutes to keep good and moist. Serves 4–6.

*Note:* This is fine for the family as well as someone on a semi-soft diet. By adding a little more soup to the blender first and then a portion of the meat with cheese mixture, it could also be used for a liquefied diet. A blended vegetable and potato could be added for a complete meal. Also, extra portions could be blended at the same time and placed in TV trays for the freezer, for future use on a busy day, or to take visiting or vacationing.

## CORN AND WIENER ROAST

2 tablespoons prepared mustard
2 cans (16 ounces each) cream-style corn
8 frankfurters
4 slices processed cheese
2 tablespoons butter or margarine

Preheat oven to 350° F.

In baking dish, stir prepared mustard into corn. Stuff each frankfurter with a ½ slice processed cheese by slitting entire length of frankfurter. Place on top of corn and dot corn with 2 tablespoons of butter or margarine. Bake, covered, at 350° F. for approximately 20 minutes. Serves 5–6.

*Note:* This recipe could also be made in your covered frying pan, electric frying pan, or skillet. This should be moist enough for most people on a semi-soft diet, and is an excellent one-dish meal for a liquid diet. Just add a little milk to the blender first.

## FRANKS—FAMILY STYLE

½ cup chopped onion
2 tablespoons butter or margarine
1 can Cheddar cheese soup
⅓ can milk
4 cups sliced cooked potatoes
Salt and pepper to taste
8 frankfurters—sliced diagonally

Preheat oven to 350° F.

In saucepan, cook onion in butter or margarine until tender. Stir in Cheddar cheese soup with milk to rinse out can. In baking dish, alternate cooked potatoes, sprinkled with salt and pepper, with soup mixture. Top with frankfurters. Bake covered at 350° F. for 30 minutes. Serves 5–6.

*Note:* By covering the baking dish, this meal should be moist enough for almost everyone on a semi-soft diet. For blending, add a little milk first, and then whatever portion of the meal is required. This is another excellent meal for a liquefied diet, as the ingredients in recipe give a well-balanced one-dish meal.

## FRANK 'N POTATO CASSEROLE

1 can cream of celery soup
¾ cup milk
¼ cup finely chopped onion
3 teaspoons prepared mustard
4 cups diced cooked potatoes (canned potatoes can be substituted)
Salt and pepper to taste
6 frankfurters, slit lengthwise

Preheat oven to 400° F.

In saucepan combine cream of celery soup, milk, chopped onion, and prepared mustard; simmer for 5 minutes, stirring occasionally until well mixed. In buttered 1½-quart casserole arrange alternate layers of potatoes, sprinkled with salt and pepper, 6 slit frankfurters and sauce, ending with sauce on the top layer. Bake covered at 400° F. for 40–45 minutes. Makes 4–5 servings.

*Note:* This meal could also be prepared and cooked in your frying pan or a skillet, covered, at low heat for about the same length of time. For blending, add extra milk to the blender before food. This is another good one-dish meal.

## SOUP-KETTLE SUPPER

8 frankfurters, cut into ½-inch slices
2 tablespoons margarine or butter
¼ teaspoon thyme
1 can split pea with ham soup
1 can cream of potato soup
1½ cans water
1 cup cooked whole-kernel corn
½ cup chopped tomatoes, canned or fresh

In large saucepan brown frankfurters in margarine or butter, with thyme. Add split pea with ham soup and cream of potato soup, rinsing out cans with 1½ cans water, stirring in water gradually. Continue to cook over low heat while stirring in water. Add corn and tomatoes. Heat through, stirring now and then. Makes 5–6 servings.

*Note:* This is a well-balanced nutritious meal and can be eaten by the whole family as well as by most anyone on a semi-soft diet. It can also be blended, and extra portions may be blended and frozen for future use. Because of the combined amount of vegetables plus meat in this recipe, it makes a particularly good meal for a liquid diet.

## HAM SLICE WITH CREAM OF MUSHROOM SOUP

1 ready-cooked ham slice, approximately ½ inch thick
1 can cream of mushroom soup
⅓ cup milk

Place ham slice in frying pan. Cover with cream of mushroom soup, rinsing out can with ⅓ cup of milk (water if desired). Stir soup and milk together well, cover, and simmer slowly until heated through. Serves 2–3.

*Note:* Anyone in the family can eat this, even one on a semi-soft diet; just cut meat into very small pieces and be sure it is adequately covered with the soup. For blending, just add extra milk to the blender first before adding meat and soup mixture, again being sure to cut the meat into small pieces. This places a lighter load on your blender. A portion of blended vegetable could be added to make a balanced meal.

## HAM AND CHEESE ON RYE

6 servings of sliced ham
6 slices pineapple
2 tablespoons butter or margarine
1 can Cheddar cheese soup
6 slices rye bread, toasted or plain

In frying pan at medium heat, brown ham and pineapple in butter or margarine. Meanwhile, in saucepan, pour contents of can of Cheddar cheese soup; stir gently. Top each bread slice with ham and pineapple. Pour heated soup over each. Makes 6 open-faced sandwiches.

*Note:* This recipe can be eaten by all the family and should be soft enough with the hot soup for anyone on a semi-soft diet to be able to eat it as is. However, soft white bread may be substituted, or a soft white bun. The above mixture without the bread could be blended into liquid form and served with a blended vegetable to make a balanced meal.

## OLD-FASHIONED BOILED DINNER WITH DAISY HAM

1 Daisy Ham, according to size of family
1 teaspoon parsley flakes
1 teaspoon celery flakes
Salt and pepper to taste
Dash chili powder
1 bunch carrots
4 medium potatoes (amount optional)
1 medium head cabbage

Remove outer wrappings from Daisy Ham, place in large pot, cover with water, and bring to boil. Boil approximately 10 minutes, then pour off water. Cover ham again with fresh water, bring to boil again, and reduce to low heat. Add parsley flakes, celery flakes, salt and pepper to taste, and a dash of chili powder; stir. Meanwhile, peel carrots and potatoes and cut cabbage into quarters, removing hard inner core from each. After ham has simmered for about 1 hour, add carrots and potatoes and simmer for another hour. The last 20 minutes or so, add cabbage and cook until vegetables are well done and meat is tender. A Daisy Ham about 3 pounds in size will serve 4–5.

*Note:* Daisy Ham cooked this way is very moist and tender, and can readily be eaten by anyone on a semi-soft diet by cutting meat into small pieces. Butter or margarine may be added to potatoes and carrots to make more moist and easily swallowed. For blending, all of the above except the cabbage could be blended together with some of the liquid to make the proper consistency. This is another good one-dish meal, making the work load easier on the cook!

## OVEN-COOKED CANNED HAM

3–5 pound canned ham
1 tablespoon prepared mustard
½ cup brown sugar
Large sheet heavy aluminum foil to wrap entire ham

Preheat oven to 350° F.

Open canned ham and place in center of sheet of heavy aluminum foil on baking dish. Add prepared mustard to brown sugar and mix well. Pour over top of ham and fold aluminum foil across the top and on each side. Bake at 350° F. for approximately 1 hour, or until heated through. Serves 5–6.

*Note:* This method of baking ham, as with the roast beef, makes it much more tender and juicy. The entire family can eat it and it can also be readily used for a semi-soft diet by cutting into small pieces. It can also be blended by adding the juices left in the aluminum foil to the blender first, and then adding the cut-up pieces of ham. Add a blended vegetable and potato to make a complete meal. Here again extra portions could be blended and frozen for future use in TV trays or freezer containers.

## BOUNTIFUL HARVEST SPICED HAM

⅔ cup catsup or chili sauce
⅓ cup water
1 tablespoon grated onion
⅓ cup chopped sweet pickles, or pickle relish
1 can luncheon meat

In medium-size saucepan, combine catsup or chili sauce, water, grated onion, and chopped sweet pickles or pickle relish. Open can of luncheon meat and place entire piece in saucepan and simmer, covered, about 25 minutes, or until thoroughly heated. Baste frequently and add more water if necessary. Slice and serve with sauce. Makes approximately 4 servings.

*Note:* Luncheon meat is soft and makes an ideal meal for a semi-soft diet. If the family does not care to eat this meal you could make the whole thing for the patient and freeze ahead in portions according to his appetite, either as is or blended. Just be sure to add extra liquid to the blender before adding the meat.

## MACARONI AND CHEESE WITH MEAT

1 cup luncheon meat, cubed
2 tablespoons butter or margarine
1 can (15 ounces) macaroni and cheese
1 can (8 ounces) asparagus cuts

In medium saucepan, brown luncheon meat lightly in butter or margarine. Add macaroni and cheese and asparagus cuts, stirring until thoroughly mixed, and heat through. Makes 2–3 servings.

*Note:* This meal can be chewed and swallowed easily by anyone on a semi-soft diet. However, if blending is required, add a little milk to blender first to make more liquefied.

If patient does not care for asparagus, another green vegetable may be substituted, giving a well-balanced meal in one dish.

This is a good recipe to use in your thermos bottle if you want to make a day trip, or plan to drive on a long enough trip to require a meal to be carried; even for visiting. It is an excellent one-dish meal and contains all ingredients required for a balanced diet.

## SCALLOPED HAM AND POTATOES

3 medium potatoes, sliced thin
1 medium onion, sliced thin
2 cups diced or sliced leftover ham
Salt and pepper to taste
1 can cream of mushroom soup
½–¾ can water or milk (or half and half)
1 teaspoon parsley flakes
1 teaspoon celery flakes
Dash chili powder

Preheat oven to 350° F.

In alternating layers in 1½-quart casserole dish, place potatoes, onion, and meat cut into bite-size pieces or slices, adding a little salt and pepper on potato layers, according to taste. In saucepan turn out contents of can of cream of mushroom soup, rinsing with water or milk (or half and half), adding parsley flakes, celery flakes, and chili powder, and stir until completely heated through. Pour over contents of casserole dish and bake in 350° F. oven, covered, about ¾ hour. Serves 4–5.

*Note:* Cheddar cheese soup may be substituted in this recipe—just eliminate the onion slices. This is fine for the family as well as for a semi-soft diet. By adding sufficient soup mixture to blender before adding meat and potatoes, it can also be used for a blended diet.

## VENETIAN CASSEROLE

1 can luncheon meat, cubed
1 can minestrone soup
½ cup water
1 cup canned lima beans (or fresh cooked)
2 tablespoons grated Parmesan cheese

Preheat oven to 350° F.

In 1½-quart casserole place luncheon meat, together with minestrone soup, water, and lima beans. Mix well. Add Parmesan cheese, sprinkled lightly over top. Bake covered at 350° F. 20–30 minutes, until heated through. Serves 3–4.

*Note:* This meal can be served to the family as is, as well as anyone on a semi-soft diet. If blending is required, be sure to use enough of the liquid to get the proper consistency necessary. Here again we have a good nutritious one-dish meal that could also be poured into a thermos to take with you on a trip or for visiting, making reheating unnecessary.

## ONE-DISH LAMB DINNER

4 loin lamb chops
1 tablespoon salad oil
1 can mushroom gravy
3 medium potatoes, sliced
1 teaspoon salt
½ teaspoon pepper
1 can (8½ ounces) peas or peas and carrots

In frying pan, brown lamb chops lightly in salad oil; remove excess oil. Add mushroom gravy, potatoes, salt, and pepper; stir well and simmer slowly approximately 1 hour, or until chops are tender. Add peas, or peas and carrots and simmer 2 or 3 minutes longer until vegetable is heated through. Serves 2–3.

*Note:* This can be served on a semi-soft diet, if chops are good and tender and moist, by cutting into very small pieces and adding extra gravy.

It is also an excellent one-dish nutritious meal for a liquefied diet. Just be sure to add extra gravy to blender before adding cut-up meat, potato, and vegetable.

## CREAMY PORK STEAK SUPPER

4 pork steaks
1 tablespoon salad oil
1 small onion, chopped
1 can cream of mushroom soup
½ – ¾ can milk
2 medium potatoes, sliced
1 teaspoon salt
½ teaspoon pepper

In frying pan, brown pork steaks lightly in salad oil, together with onion. Add contents of can of cream of mushroom soup together with ½ – ¾ can milk to rinse out can; stir well together. After soup mixture is well blended, add potatoes, salt, and pepper; stir. Simmer slowly, covered, approximately 50–60 minutes, until meat is very tender. Serves 2–3.

*Note:* For a semi-soft diet, just be sure meat is cut into small pieces and plenty of soup mixture is added for easy chewing and swallowing. If blending is necessary, add enough soup mixture to blender before adding cut-up meat and potatoes. Extra milk can be added if more liquid consistency is necessary. Add a blended vegetable for a balanced meal, if desired.

## PORK AND VEGETABLE MEDLEY

4 pork steaks, ½–¾ inch thick
2 tablespoons salad oil
1 cup chopped onion
¼ medium head cabbage, shredded
4 medium potatoes, sliced
1½ teaspoons salt
½ teaspoon pepper
1 can cream of asparagus soup
½ can milk

In frying pan brown pork steaks lightly in salad oil. Set aside and pour off any excess fat. After steaks have been set aside and excess fat poured off, in the same frying pan combine onion, cabbage, potatoes, salt, and pepper, together with cream of asparagus soup. Use milk to rinse out can and add to this mixture; stir thoroughly. Replace pork steaks in frying pan, cover, and simmer approximately 1 hour, or until well done and tender. Baste occasionally. More milk can be added if desired. Serves 3–4.

*Note:* This can be eaten by everyone, even on a semi-soft diet, if kept good and moist. It can also be blended as well, just being sure enough soup mixture is added to blender first, making still another easy meal for the cook, being a one-dish meal. Always remember, the more liquid added to the blender, the thinner the consistency of the food.

## ITALIANO STEAK

2 tablespoons salad oil
1 pound top round steak, ½ inch thick
1 can tomato soup
½ can water
1 can (2 ounces) sliced mushrooms, drained
1 clove garlic, minced
1 teaspoon orégano, crushed
Salt and pepper to taste

Warm 2 tablespoons salad oil in frying pan and brown steak, cut into serving-size pieces, lightly. Pour off any excess fat. Stir in remaining ingredients: tomato soup, water to rinse can, mushrooms, garlic, orégano, and salt and pepper to taste. Cover, stirring occasionally and cook over low simmer 1 hour, or until tender. Serves 2–3.

*Note:* This is an excellent recipe for the whole family, and more ingredients may be added according to the size of the family. You can also add slices of potato, making a balanced meal. If you use a good cut of steak and cut it into small pieces, anyone on a semi-soft diet should have no difficulty swallowing, as it is very tender and moist. If blending is required, be sure to put enough of the tomato soup into the blender first before the rest of the ingredients (more water may be added if additional liquid is desired). Also, be sure to cut the meat into small pieces as this places less of a strain on the blender motor.

## STEAK WITH ONION SOUP

2 tablespoons salad oil
1 pound top round steak, ½ inch thick
1 can onion soup
½ cup catsup
Salt and pepper to taste
1 medium green pepper, cut into thin strips

In frying pan warm salad oil and lightly brown steak, cut into serving-size pieces; pour off any excess fat. Add onion soup, catsup, and salt and pepper to taste. Simmer slowly about 40 minutes; add green pepper strips and simmer about 20 minutes more, or until meat and vegetable are tender. Stir now and then and baste steak. Serves 2–3.

*Note:* This is an excellent recipe for the whole family, and more ingredients may be added according to the size of the family. You can also add slices of potato, making a balanced meal. If you use a good cut of steak and cut it into small pieces, anyone on a semi-soft diet should have no difficulty swallowing, as it is very tender and moist. If blending is required, be sure to put enough of the onion soup into the blender first before adding the rest of the ingredients (more water may be added if additional liquifaction is desired). Be sure to cut the meat into small pieces as this places less of a strain on the blender motor. If you plan to use this recipe for a blended diet, a cheaper cut of chuck steak could be substituted, making it a little easier on the pocketbook!

## STEAK WITH VEGETABLE SOUP

1 pound top round steak, ½ inch thick
2 tablespoons salad oil
1 can vegetable soup
½ can water
1 cup sliced onion
Salt and pepper to taste

Cut steak into serving-size portions and brown lightly in salad oil in frying pan; pour off any excess fat. Add vegetable soup, water to rinse out can (more water may be added if desired), onion, salt and pepper to taste. Mix well. Cover and simmer on low heat for 1 hour, or until good and tender.

*Note:* This recipe could be enjoyed by all the family, and slices of potato could be added, making a balanced meal. If you use a good cut of meat and cut it into small pieces, anyone on a semi-soft diet should have no difficulty swallowing, as it is very tender and moist. Where blending is necessary, be sure to add enough vegetable soup first before adding the rest of the ingredients to the blender. More water may be added if additional liquid is desired. Chuck steak, for a blended diet would work out fine, thus saving money—something we all enjoy these days!

## ROAST VEAL

4–5 pound veal roast
Salt and pepper to taste
¼ teaspoon thyme
¼ teaspoon rosemary
4 medium sweet potatoes, for baking

Preheat oven to 325° F.

Wipe roast with damp cloth. Place in roasting pan and sprinkle with salt and pepper to taste, thyme, and rosemary. Bake uncovered in slow oven (325° F.) about 40 minutes per pound. Put sweet potatoes to bake in oven at the same time. Be sure to save juices from roasting pan to make gravy, or use canned gravy if desired. Serves 4–5.

*Note:* This can be served readily for the family, and for anyone on a semi-soft diet, just cut meat into small pieces and cover with gravy. Sweet potatoes can be made more moist and easy to swallow by adding butter or margarine. If blending is required, just be sure to add gravy to blender first and then the cut-up pieces of meat.

Sweet potatoes in a can could be substituted and could also be blended if required by adding milk and butter.

# *Poultry*

## CHICKEN DIVINE

1 package frozen broccoli
4–6 chicken steaks
1 teaspoon salt
½ teaspoon pepper
1 can cream of mushroom soup

Preheat oven to 350° F.
Cook broccoli, drain. Place in bottom of casserole dish and arrange 4–6 chicken steaks on top of the broccoli. Sprinkle salt and pepper over all. Cover chicken steaks and broccoli entirely with contents of can of cream of mushroom soup (¼–½ can milk may be added if more moisture is desired). Bake covered at 350° F. about 40 minutes. Serves 3–4.

*Note:* This is a particularly tasty dish and certainly can be eaten by everyone in the family, as well as one on a semi-soft diet. For a liquefied diet, add extra milk to the blender first before placing portion of chicken steaks and broccoli desired by patient. It can be used as a one-dish meal for a blended diet, as it contains poultry, vegetable, and protein.

## CREAMED CHICKEN LEGS

4 chicken legs
2 tablespoons shortening
Salt and pepper to taste
1 can cream of chicken soup
½–¾ can water or milk
1 large potato, sliced thin

In heavy skillet or frying pan, brown chicken legs lightly in shortening; pour off any excess fat. Salt and pepper to taste. Pour contents of can of cream of chicken soup, rinsed out with milk or water, over chicken legs. Place slices of potato in soup around chicken legs, cover, and simmer slowly approximately 1 hour, or until tender. Serves 3–4.

*Note:* This is another excellent meal for the whole family as well as one on a semi-soft diet. Just cut meat off the chicken legs and add sufficient liquid over meat and potato slices so it can easily be chewed and swallowed. For blending, just before serving the family, remove skin from chicken leg, cut meat, add some of the soup mixture to the blender first, and then the cut-up chicken and a few potato slices. More milk can be added if a more liquefied mixture is desired.

# Seafood

## CREAMED TUNA FISH AND PEAS

1 can (7 ounces) tuna fish
1 small onion, diced
¼ cup flour
1 can (14½ ounces) evaporated milk
1 can (1 pound) peas

Drain oil from tuna fish into saucepan. Add onion and cook over low heat until tender. Remove from heat. Stir in flour—then gradually add evaporated milk, continuing to stir. Drain liquid from peas into evaporated milk mixture and stir.

Return to heat, cook stirring constantly about 10 minutes. Add contents of can of tuna fish, flaked, with peas and continue stirring and cooking slowly until hot and thickened.

Serve on light toast, mashed potatoes, rice, or noodles. Makes approximately 6 servings.

*Note:* Everyone in the family, as well as anyone on a semi-soft diet can eat this as is. For blending, pour extra milk into the blender first before adding portion of food required by the patient.

## CURRIED TUNA FISH

1 can cream of mushroom soup
⅓ cup milk
1 teaspoon curry (celery salt or parlsey flakes may be substituted)
1 can (7 ounces) tuna fish

Empty contents of can of cream of mushroom soup into saucepan, together with milk used to rinse out can. Add curry (or substitute) and tuna fish, drained and flaked.

Stir entire mixture over medium heat until hot and well mixed. Serve on toast, English muffins or hamburger rolls. Serves 2–3.

*Note:* This can readily be eaten by everyone in the family as well as anyone on a semi-soft diet, in which case soft bread or hamburger rolls would be easier for him to swallow. It also blends very well—just add a little extra milk to the blender first, making a very nutritious meal for anyone needing a completely liquefied diet. This also could be carried along in a thermos for an outing or visit.

## CELERY-SALMON LOAF

1 can (1 pound) salmon with juice, flaked
1½ cups dry bread crumbs
½ cup minced green pepper
2 eggs, slightly beaten
1 can cream of celery soup

Preheat oven to 350° F.

In mixing bowl combine the following ingredients and mix well: salmon, bread crumbs, green pepper, eggs, and can of cream of celery soup. Pack this mixture into a greased loaf pan and bake for about 1 hour at 350° F., or until done. Pour off extra juices and serve on a warm platter. While this is baking, make the following celery sauce to place over salmon loaf before serving:

**Celery Sauce**

1 can cream of celery soup
1 teaspoon prepared mustard
¼ cup milk
3 tablespoons sweet pickle relish
1 hard-cooked egg, chopped

Empty contents of can of cream of celery soup into saucepan; blend in prepared mustard and milk, used to rinse out can. Add sweet pickle relish and hard-cooked egg. Stir over low heat until well blended, and pour over salmon loaf, which has been placed on a warm platter. Serves 5–6.

*Note:* This is good for all the family and very soft and moist for anyone on a semi-soft diet. If it is felt that the celery bits in the soup might be hard to swallow, just blend the soup first before using in recipe. This can also be used for a blended diet by adding extra sauce and milk to the blender first to get the proper consistency.

## QUICK SEAFOOD DELIGHT

1 package (1½ cups) Minute Rice
2 tablespoons butter or margarine
⅓ cup catsup
4 drops Tabasco sauce
1 teaspoon Worcestershire sauce
¾ teaspoon salt
1½ cups light cream
1½ cups water
1 can (7 ounces) shrimp (crab meat may be substituted)

In frying pan or heavy skillet, sauté Minute Rice in butter or margarine, at low simmer. Add catsup, Tabasco sauce, Worcestershire sauce, salt, light cream, and water. Blend well with fork, bring to boil, uncovered, fluffing once or twice. (Do not stir.) Cover and simmer at low heat for 10 minutes. Add shrimp and heat 1 minute longer or until thoroughly heated through. Serves 4–5.

*Note:* This is a very tasty meal and should be enjoyed by the whole family, as well as anyone on a semi-soft diet. If necessary, additional cream or water could be added should more moisture be desired. It can also be blended by adding extra milk to the blender first to make the proper consistency.

## SHRIMP CREOLE

¼ cup finely chopped onion
¼ cup finely chopped green pepper
2 tablespoons salad oil
1 can tomato soup
½ can water
1 teaspoon vinegar
Dash Tabasco sauce
Dash black pepper
1 pound frozen or fresh shrimp, cooked
3 cups cooked rice

In frying pan sauté onion and green pepper in salad oil until soft. Add tomato soup with water to rinse out can, stir, and add vinegar, Tabasco sauce, and black pepper. Cook over low simmer about 10 minutes, stirring occasionally. Add shrimp and simmer 5 minutes longer. Place hot cooked rice on warm serving dish and pour shrimp mixture on top of rice. Makes approximately 6 servings.

*Note:* This is very tasty and nutritious and can readily be eaten by someone on a semi-soft diet, as well as enjoyed by the whole family. However, if the rice cannot be swallowed easily, creamy mashed potatoes could be substituted. This can also be blended by adding extra water or tomato soup to the blender for proper consistency, using just the shrimp mixture. Add a blended vegetable and potato for a balanced meal.

## SHRIMP 'N NEWBURG SAUCE

1 can (10½ ounces) Newburg sauce
1 can (4½ ounces) tiny cocktail shrimp, drained

In medium-size saucepan, empty contents of can of Newburg sauce. Drain shrimp and add to Newburg sauce, stirring well until heated through. Serve on toast, soft bread, or open-faced rolls. Serves 2–3.

*Note:* This is an excellent "quick dish" meal and can be used for a semi-soft diet as well as for the family. Tuna fish, crab meat, or lobster could be substituted. If blending is necessary, add extra milk to the blender first for additional moisture. However, if lobster is used, do not blend.

# Vegetables

### BROCCOLI WITH CHICKEN CREAM SAUCE

1 can cream of chicken soup
⅓ cup milk
1 pound broccoli, cooked and drained (frozen may be used)

Empty contents of can of cream of chicken soup into small saucepan, stir in milk, and simmer about 2 minutes. Cook and drain broccoli, either fresh or frozen. Place drained broccoli on serving dish and pour contents of saucepan over all.

*Note:* This can easily be eaten by anyone on a semi-soft diet and could be an entire meal for anyone on a blended diet, with the bits of chicken that are in the soup. Just add a little extra milk to blender first.

## SCALLOPED POTATOES

4 medium potatoes, peeled and sliced
2 tablespoons butter or margarine
2 tablespoons flour
1 teaspoon salt
1½–2 cups milk
¾ cup American or Cheddar cheese, cut up

Preheat oven to 375° F.

Arrange potatoes in bottom of baking dish. In saucepan, melt butter or margarine, add flour and salt and mix well. Add milk. When sauce is thick, add cheese, stirring frequently.

Remove from heat and immediately pour over potatoes which have already been arranged in baking dish. Bake at 375° F. about 1 hour. Serves 4.

*Note:* By adding extra milk to the blender first, this recipe could be liquefied enough for a patient needing only blended foods.

## Chapter 4

# DESSERTS

## General Information

This chapter contains dessert recipes that almost anyone can eat, either semi-soft or blended, as well as the whole family. Included too are a few fancy desserts for that extra special occasion to lift the spirits.

Some people have a sweet tooth, and to them, a dessert can be a real treat. If their appetites are not too good, and a sweet appeals to them, you can find some particularly nourishing recipes that they like and serve to them between meals. Adding whipped cream or any whipped topping might also tempt them.

If blended food is required, save some of your energy by blending larger portions at one time and storing the extra food in the refrigerator or freezer. Having to use the blender every couple of hours, thereby necessitating the washing of same, can get to be a real annoyance, and let's avoid that by all means!

There are also many packaged puddings, Jell-O, and prepared egg custard desserts that you can obtain at your local supermarkets. The puddings and egg custard usually require milk to be added, and for extra nutrition, you can use the fortified milk explained in Chapter 5.

Canned and frozen fruits are a great convenience—the only work being involved is a can opener! For a semi-soft diet they could be used as is, or added to ice cream. If a liquefied diet is required, simply turn the entire contents of the can or frozen package (thawed, of course!) into the blender and serve in quantities desired. Extra portions may be stored for future use. The use of fruit is a change of pace, plus contributing to a well-balanced meal.

Just plain ice cream always makes a good dessert and can be dressed up, according to the patient's ability to chew or swallow, by adding fruit or whipped topping. If the patient has difficulty swallowing, place a scoop or two in a sauce dish ½ hour or so before serving, and when it softens enough, stir until of liquid consistency.

This could also apply to people who have the problem of not being able to stand extremes of too hot or too cold food—allowing the ice cream to reach room temperature makes the ice cream more palatable for them.

## LIME-APPLE FROST

1¼ cups applesauce
1 package lime-flavored gelatin
¾ cup sugar
1 cup evaporated milk (very cold)
1 tablespoon lime or lemon juice

In saucepan, heat applesauce to boiling; add lime-flavored gelatin, stirring until dissolved. Mix in sugar and cook until almost stiff.

In separate mixing bowl, whip evaporated milk with lime or lemon juice until stiff. Add to gelatin mixture and beat in slowly. Place in mold or dessert dishes. Chill at least 1 hour. Serve with whipped cream or whipped topping already prepared. Makes approximately 4–5 servings.

*Note:* This makes a very smooth dessert and, with evaporated milk being used, also gives extra nutrition. This could be eaten by the family as well as anyone on a semi-soft diet. By adding a little extra milk to the blender, it could be liquefied to the consistency desired.

## APRICOT WHIP

1 envelope unflavored gelatin
¼ cup cold water
¼ cup sugar
¼ teaspoon salt
½ cup hot apricot syrup or hot water
1 cup mashed canned apricots
2 tablespoons lemon juice
2 egg whites, stiffly beaten
Apricot halves, optional

In mixing bowl, soften gelatin in cold water; add sugar, salt, and hot apricot syrup or hot water, and stir until completely dissolved. Add mashed apricots (or blended) and lemon juice. Chill in refrigerator and, when mixture begins to thicken, fold in egg whites. Turn into mold that has been rinsed in cold water, and chill until firm. When completely firm, unmold onto serving dish and garnish with apricot halves, if desired. For added garnishment, a bit of whipped cream or whipped topping could be dropped into each apricot half.

*Note:* This is something almost anyone can eat. If a blended diet is necessary, leave the apricot half off the patient's portion and garnish with cream alone if he likes.

## BREAD PUDDING

1½ cups light brown sugar
1 tablespoon butter or margarine
4 slices soft white bread, generously buttered and cut into cubes
3 eggs
2½ cups milk
1 teaspoon vanilla
¼ teaspoon salt

Preheat oven to 350° F.

Melt and mix well light brown sugar and butter or margarine in top of double boiler. Pour into medium-size casserole baking dish and add bread. In separate bowl combine eggs, milk, vanilla, and salt, and beat well. Pour over bread, but *do not* stir. Place in pan of water and bake in oven at 350° F. for 1 hour. Serves 6.

*Note:* This is very moist and should be easily swallowed. This could be blended also by adding extra milk to the blender first, adding more if necessary to make more liquefied.

# *Creamy Type Puddings*

## CREAM TAPIOCA PUDDING

1 egg, separated
4 tablespoons sugar
2 cups milk
4 tablespoons tapioca
⅛ teaspoon salt
½ teaspoon vanilla, or extract of your choice

Beat white of egg with egg beater or blender, adding 2 tablespoons sugar, one at a time; continue until it stands in peaks and set aside. Mix yolk of egg with ½ cup milk in saucepan, stir well. Add tapioca, 2 tablespoons sugar, and salt; mix again and then add the other 1½ cups of the milk. Place over low heat and cook until mixture comes to a boil, about 5–7 minutes. Stir constantly. Does not have to cook until completely thick for it will thicken as it cools. Do not overcook, just let boil a few minutes. Remove from heat and stir in the beaten egg white set aside, and add ½ teaspoon vanilla or extract of your choice.

*Note:* Almost anyone could eat this except possibly someone on a strictly liquid diet. However, if he enjoys it, just add extra milk to your blender and a portion of the pudding, blending to the consistency desired.

## FLOATING ISLAND DELUXE

2 cups milk
2 tablespoons salad oil
¼ cup sugar
1 tablespoon cornstarch
⅛ teaspoon salt
3 tablespoons cocoa
2 eggs, separated
½ teaspoon vanilla

Pour milk into saucepan and scald. In separate bowl mix salad oil with sugar, cornstarch, salt, cocoa, and mix well. Add egg yolks, slightly beaten. Add scalded milk slowly to egg mixture, stirring constantly. Cook in top of double boiler until mixture coats spoon, stirring constantly. Cool. Add vanilla. Serve hilled, topped with whipped cream or with peaks of uncooked meringue (made by beating 2 egg whites stiff with ¼ cup sugar). Makes 4–6 servings.

*Note:* Almost everyone should be able to eat this, except maybe someone on a completely liquid diet. But, as with the tapioca pudding, extra milk could be added to your blender first and then a portion of the pudding, blended to the desired consistency.

## HAVANA BANANA CREAM PUDDING

1 egg, separated
4 cups milk
⅓ cup Minute Tapioca
½ cup sugar
¼ teaspoon salt
1 teaspoon vanilla
2 bananas, diced

In saucepan mix egg yolk with a small amount of milk over low heat, enough to blend the two together well. Add tapioca, sugar, salt, and the remainder of the milk. Bring quickly to a full boil, stirring constantly. Remove from heat. (Mixture will be thick. Do not overcook.) Beat egg white until just stiff enough to hold shape. Fold into hot tapioca mixture gradually. Cool—mixture again thickens as it cools. When slightly cool, stir in vanilla and chill. Just before serving, fold bananas into chilled mixture. Garnish with banana slices if desired or with whipped cream. Makes approximately 8 servings.

*Note:* As with other creamy puddings, practically everyone should be able to eat this one too, except for someone on a completely liquid diet. To liquefy, just add extra milk to blender before adding portion of pudding.

## ORANGE BAVARIAN CREAM PUDDING

1 tablespoon unflavored gelatin
¼ cup cold water
¾ cup unstrained orange juice
2 tablespoons lemon juice
½ teaspoon grated orange rind
⅓ cup sugar
¼ teaspoon salt
1 egg white
½ cup cream, whipped

Sprinkle gelatin on cold water and let soak a few minutes in small bowl. In saucepan, heat unstrained orange juice, lemon juice, and grated orange rind with half the sugar listed above. Add dissolved gelatin to hot juices and chill in refrigerator until partly set. In separate bowl, add salt to egg white and beat until stiff. Add the remaining half of the sugar slowly, beating until glossy. Fold egg white mixture and ½ cup whipped cream into gelatin mixture. Pour into mold and chill until firm. Serves 3–4.

*Note:* The unstrained orange juice and grated orange rind might make this difficult for some people to swallow. If so, both items could be blended before making the recipe. For a liquefied diet, just add extra milk or cream for the proper consistency.

## WHIPPED MOCHA MIST

1 tablespoon unflavored gelatin
1 package (4 ounces) butterscotch pudding
1½ teaspoons instant coffee
¼ cup sugar
1⅔ cups evaporated milk
2 tablespoons orange juice

In saucepan mix gelatin, butterscotch pudding, instant coffee, sugar, and 1 cup of the evaporated milk. Cook over low heat until mixture comes to a full boil, stirring constantly. Chill in refrigerator until mixture mounds from spoon. While mixing the above, chill ⅔ cup evaporated milk in freezer in ice-cube tray until soft ice crystals form around edges of tray (10–15 minutes). Remove and scoop into mixing bowl and beat until stiff, about 1 minute; add orange juice and beat again until very stiff, about 2 minutes longer. Add to pudding mixture and beat well. Spoon into sherbet or parfait glasses and chill until firm, about 2 hours. Garnish with whipped cream or whipped topping if desired. Serves 4–5.

*Note:* Almost anyone can eat this without trouble except for someone on a liquefied diet but this can still be used for that by adding extra milk to the blender first for extra moisture.

## PEACH CREAM DESSERT

1 package (4 ounces) vanilla pudding
1 pint milk
1 can (16 ounces) sliced yellow cling peaches

In saucepan, make vanilla pudding according to directions. Pour off juice from can of peaches and arrange slices on pie plate or in shallow mold. Pour cooled pudding over slices and chill thoroughly. Serve as is or with whipped cream or whipped topping. Serves 3–4.

*Note:* This can be eaten by all the family as well as someone on a semi-soft diet. Use additional milk or some of the peach juice in the blender for a liquefied diet.

## LEMON CHIFFON DESSERT

1 package (4–4½ ounces) lemon chiffon pie filling
½ cup boiling water
1 can (1 pound) fruit cocktail
¼ cup sugar
2 tablespoons lemon juice
1 cup finely crushed graham cracker crumbs

Turn contents of package of lemon chiffon pie filling into large bowl of electric mixer or regular mixing bowl. Add boiling water and mix thoroughly. Drain ½ cup syrup from large can of fruit cocktail and add to lemon chiffon mix. Beat with electric mixer or rotary beater until very foamy, about 1 minute. Add sugar and continue beating until mixture stands in very stiff peaks. Fold in lemon juice and well-drained contents of can of fruit cocktail. Sprinkle ¾ cup fine graham cracker crumbs in bottom of 8-inch-square pan and then pour contents of mixing bowl over crumbs. Sprinkle top with additional ¼ cup of crumbs if desired. Chill until firm, then cut into squares to serve. Makes 9 servings.

*Note:* If the patient finds the graham cracker crumbs too hard to swallow, eliminate this step of the recipe. Instead, a mold may be used or the mixture just placed in individual dessert dishes. Whipped cream or whipped topping could be used for decoration. For a liquefied diet add some of the syrup from the can of fruit cocktail to the blender first and then a portion of dessert and blend to desired consistency.

## MELON RINGS WITH STRAWBERRIES

1 medium melon
1 package frozen strawberries, thawed

Cut melon crosswise into rings 1 inch thick; remove seeds. Place slices on plate. With knife, loosen pulp by cutting around slice ¼ inch from rind—do not remove rind. Slice pulp to make bite-size pieces, leaving rind intact. Mix bite-size pieces of melon with strawberries and arrange in center of each slice. Serves 5–6.

*Note:* If patient should find this difficult to swallow, the strawberries and bite-size pieces of melon can be blended and placed in the center of each slice. If desired, whipped topping or whipped cream can be added on top of each mound to make more attractive-looking. This is one of the desserts mentioned that could be used for a festive occasion. It is not a great deal of work, but is attractive-looking and light, as well as nutritious.

## Chapter 5

# EXTRA NUTRITION

## General Information

For various reasons, some people have a poor appetite or are unable to eat normal-size meals, thereby requiring extra nutrition in what they can manage to eat. Rather than trying to force too much on them, which causes an even more anti-eating feeling (plus irritation!), you might follow some helpful suggestions in this chapter.

Included here are ideas for getting this extra nutrition into the patient without increasing the amount of food or liquid intake. There are also some recipes containing evaporated milk, which also gives extra food value. If the family does not care for some of these meals, on a day when you have a little free time, prepare the entire recipes and place the extra portions in freezer containers for future use.

To put extra nutrition into the milk they consume, add 1 cup of dry powdered milk to each quart of milk, mixing well with egg beater or blender. If large quantities of milk are used, mix or blend ½ gallon or more at one time for convenience. This milk should be used for drinking, as well as in the preparation of food requiring milk, except for those recipes calling for evaporated milk.

Eggnogs and milk shakes are further sources of extra nutrition, especially if the patient is on a blended diet or has little appetite. When there is a loss of appetite, these can be given between meals to increase the amount of food intake. Recipes for eggnog and milk shakes can be found in this chapter under Beverages. If the patient has been used to an occasional cocktail under normal conditions, you could probably tempt him into drinking an extra eggnog by adding a jigger of whiskey when blending, if permitted on his diet. This way you get the extra nutrition into him with the added bonus of this little "goody" included.

There are packages of Instant Breakfast which contain ingredients equal to a full-size breakfast. Just add a package to a glass of fortified milk and presto—a good nutritious breakfast with the minimum amount of fuss. This can be easily swallowed for a liquid diet and also is very useful on a semi-soft diet for a quick and easy meal. This is available at just about any supermarket. Available too is a drink in a can called Nutrament, which can be purchased at your drugstore or supermarket. It has the taste of a milk shake and contains extra calories and protein for those patients requiring body-building energy food. This can be used as a supplement to the regular diet, and the added treat for the cook is—no preparation!

This might prove a little on the rich side for some people, so it might be wise not to use it as a steady diet. But, as far as that is concerned—who of us wants to eat or drink the same thing every day! That's the purpose of this book—to give variety but also simplicity as much as possible for the one preparing and planning meals. You could avail yourself of this product on days when you are especially busy and don't have time to fuss.

Instant Cream of Wheat in packages, also available at your supermarket, can be diluted to a very liquefied consistency by adding butter and the above mentioned fortified milk or evaporated milk. This can be used for breakfast, but can also be utilized for a light lunch or food supplement for anyone who can eat just small amounts at a time.

Finally, try to keep a light and easy approach in trying to get the patient to eat—don't apply too much pressure—and you'll all be happier for it!

# Semi-soft Recipes

## Dairy Products

### CHEESE SOUFFLÉ

¾ teaspoon dry mustard
⅛ teaspoon cayenne pepper
1½ teaspoons sugar
½ teaspoon salt
2 teaspoons water
3 tablespoons butter
3 tablespoons sifted flour
½ cup American cheese, cut in small pieces
¾ cup milk, warmed
3 eggs, separated

Mix first four items in water.
Preheat oven to 375° F.
Melt butter in skillet over low heat. Keeping pan over low heat, mix in flour thoroughly. Add cheese cut into small pieces, slowly stirring until it partially melts and looks curdled. Then add milk very gradually, stirring mixture slowly and constantly. Continue stirring until cheese is melted and completely smooth. Add seasonings (the first

four items mixed in water). Beat egg yolks until thick and lemon-colored. Add them to cheese mixture (still over low heat) and stir until mixture is like thick custard. Remove skillet from stove.

When mixture is cool, beat the egg whites until stiff and gently fold into the cheese mixture. Now pour into a well-buttered, deep pudding dish and set in pan of water in moderate oven (375°F.). Bake for 15 minutes, then slightly increase heat to 400°F. for another 15 minutes. Soufflé will rise high and be a rich brown color when baked. Serve immediately. 6 servings.

*Note:* This is very nutritious, and almost everyone should be able to eat it. Add vegetable or salad, or blended vegetable if necessary.

### Soufflé variations:

Chicken, corn, fish, ham. Blend or place in meat grinder, whichever you desire. Follow recipe for Cheese Soufflé with one exception: In the cheese recipe the cheese has to be melted before the milk is added, but with the soufflé variations, add the meat, *then* immediately start adding the milk. Season to your own taste.

## CREAMED EGGS

2 tablespoons butter
2 tablespoons flour
1 teaspoon salt
1 can (14½ ounces) evaporated milk
4 hard-cooked eggs, sliced

Melt butter in frying pan or heavy skillet over low heat. Blend in flour and salt. Gradually stir in evaporated milk and continue simmering, stirring until thickened and smooth.

Add the hard-cooked eggs and heat a few minutes longer. Stir gently.

Serve on toast, hot cooked rice, or mashed potatoes. Makes approximately 4 servings.

*Note:* The family can eat this, as well as anyone on a semi-soft diet. If the person on the semi-soft diet should find the toast, rice, or potatoes difficult to swallow, they can just be eliminated and the eggs served as is.

# Semi-soft and Blended Recipes

## *Meats and Vegteables*

### CORNED BEEF AND VEGETABLES

3 medium potatoes, peeled and cubed
4 carrots, peeled and cubed
1 medium onion, sliced
1 cup water
¼ cup butter or margarine
¼ cup flour
½ teaspoon salt
¼ teaspoon pepper
1 can (14½ ounces) evaporated milk
1 can (12 ounces) corned beef

Place potatoes, carrots, onion, and water in large saucepan. Bring water to boil, cover pan with lid, and cook over medium-low heat until vegetables are tender—approximately 15 minutes. Stir in butter until melted. Remove from heat and stir in flour, salt, and pepper. Mix well. Slowly stir in evaporated milk.

Break corned beef into chunks with fork—add to vegetable mixture. Return to heat and cook over low heat, stirring occasionally until thickened. Makes 6 normal servings.

*Note:* This meal has extra nutrition for those people who need it for health reasons. It can be eaten by the whole family as is. If the patient needs food in liquid form, this recipe can be blended readily into the size portions he needs. Or, if the family doesn't care to eat it, the whole thing can be blended and placed in freezer containers, according to the amount he can eat. Just thaw and heat through when ready to use.

## MEAT AND GREEN BEAN CASSEROLE

¼ cup butter or margarine
2 medium onions, sliced
½ cup flour
¼ teaspoon pepper
1 can (14½ ounces) evaporated milk
1 can (1 pound) cut green beans
1 can (12 ounces) luncheon meat
1 tablespoon butter or margarine
1 slice bread

Preheat oven to 350° F.
Melt butter or margarine in saucepan over low heat. Add onions and cook until tender. Remove from heat and stir in flour and pepper. Slowly stir in evaporated milk. Add green beans with their liquid. Return to heat and cook, stirring occasionally until thickened. Cut luncheon meat into ½-inch cubes and add to bean mixture. Turn into well-greased 1½-quart baking dish.

Melt butter in small saucepan and remove from heat. Pull bread into small crumbs and add to butter, mixing lightly with fork. Spread buttered crumbs evenly over top of meat mixture in baking dish. Bake in preheated oven (350° F.) until crumbs are browned, approximately 15 minutes. Makes 6 servings.

*Note:* If the patient can eat semi-soft foods but can't eat a topping such as this recipe calls for, which might be irritating to his throat, the topping may be eliminated; or, cover dish with its own cover or with aluminum foil while baking, to retain moisture.

This could also be blended for a liquid diet by adding a little milk in the bottom of the blender first and then whatever portion the patient can eat. Add more milk if necessary to get the proper consistency.

# *Beverages*

### EGGNOG

1 egg
1 teaspoon sugar
1 cup milk
1 teaspoon vanilla extract
Dash nutmeg (optional)

Break egg and drop into blender with sugar. Blend approximately 1 minute. Add milk, vanilla, and nutmeg if desired. Makes approximately 1½ cups.

### MILK SHAKE

1 cup milk
1 scoop ice cream
1 teaspoon vanilla extract

Place milk, ice cream, and vanilla in blender and blend until foamy. Vanilla ice cream or any favorite flavor may be used. Makes 2 cups.

## Chapter 6

# PREPARED FOODS

Many food items are available in grocery stores or supermarkets for use in quick and nutritious meals, all of which are pre-cooked, either in cans or in the frozen food section, just requiring heating and serving as is, or which can be blended if a liquid diet is necessary.

## Frozen Food Department

*Complete TV Dinners:* These can sometimes be eaten as is for a semi-soft diet. If not, they can also be blended with the appropriate gravy or liquid to make the proper consistency. (Be sure to save these trays after using for making your own TV dinners—saves a few cents, and don't we all love to be able to do that today!) One dinner consisting of macaroni and cheese, peas, and apple slices can easily be eaten on a semi-soft diet. For blending, heat and add sufficient milk to the blender first to make it well liquefied. This is an excellent meal to carry in your thermos bottle if you plan a motor trip which carries you over a lunch period or any meal time, as it is very nutritious and tasty.

*Casserole Dishes:* There are a variety of this type of frozen meals merely requiring heating, and most can be used for a semi-soft diet as well as being blended after heating.

*Vegetables:* Many vegetables can be served as is with the necessary condiments or heated and blended if required. There are a few vegetables now available, and becoming more and more so, which contain other ingredients such as noodles, etc., and in some cases these could be used as a meal for someone with a poor appetite, either semi-soft as is or for a liquid diet by blending.

*Soups:* Various frozen soups can be used for a semi-soft diet by defrosting and heating through, and which also can be blended. Most of them are very nutritious and very tasty.

*Beef and Chicken Pot Pies:* These make excellent balanced meals, as they contain meat or poultry, potatoes, peas and carrots and gravy, plus the crust. They can usually be eaten by anyone on a semi-soft diet, although if the crust is too crisp, this could just be removed. When blending, just remove some of the crust, add approximately ½ can of beef or chicken gravy to the blender, then the heated pot pie, and blend until it is at the proper consistency. More or less gravy may be used as desired.

*Canned Meats:* There are various types of canned meats that can be used, as most of them are of a very soft texture, and anyone on a semi-soft diet could easily make use of them with little or no chewing and no difficulty swallowing. They also can be blended very readily. You will find many recipes utilizing many of these meats and poultry in the chapters for semi-soft and semi-soft and blended foods as well as the chapter on Extra Nutrition.

*Canned Italian Foods:* There is also a very great variety of spaghetti, macaroni, and ravioli meals with sauces and cheese or meat balls, all of which could easily be eaten on a semi-soft diet, requiring little more than just heating, which is a great help for the cook.

*Canned Vegetables:* Some of the canned vegetables could readily be used for a semi-soft diet. If blending is required, open can and turn entire contents into the blender, just adding desired condiments such as salt and pepper and butter. The same can be done with canned potatoes, either white or sweet. If a large can is used, portion-size amounts can be placed in freezer containers for future use after taking what is required for that particular meal.

*Canned Soups:* A great variety of canned soups is available, with many new ones of the heartier type coming out. Some can be used easily for a semi-soft diet, if you just add soup or milk as directed on the can. For a more liquefied diet, turn contents of can into blender, add half the can of soup or milk, blend, and then add the other half, blending well. If the patient has a poor appetite, one of the heartier soups could even be used as a main meal.

*Cheese:* There is a Welsh rarebit in a can, requiring heating only, and it can be served on toast or soft bread for a quick and easy meal. Cheese is a good protein food and should be used as often as possible to help maintain a balanced diet.

Your supermarket with its vast supply of canned and frozen foods can be your best friend and helper with a little imagination on your part.

Spend some time looking around when you shop, and you'll be amazed at the number of meals that you can utilize to make your meal planning easier!

## Chapter 7

# FREEZING AND PLANNING AHEAD

*Don't say no to visiting or vacationing!*
Just because there may be a family member with an eating problem, there is no reason to refuse invitations to eat at a friend's home, or even to take a vacation. For vacationing, the only requirements are a cooler to pack the frozen foods into while traveling and a stove to heat the meals at your destination. For traveling to your vacation spot, a thermos bottle for hot foods comes in very handy so the patient does not need skip a meal. The wide-mouth type is convenient for a semi-soft meal as well as the liquefied type. For semi-soft meals, whenever you plan a meal that is to the patient's liking, make an extra portion or two and place in freezer containers, properly marked, and leave in freezer for just such occasions—or for a day you might be extra busy and want something that needs only defrosting and heating.

If blended food is required, on a day when the person planning meals is not too busy, she should open and blend a full can of vegetables or fruit at one time, adding the necessary condiments, and place in freezer containers in meal-size portions. The canned potatoes, white or sweet, can be handled the same way.

Those aluminum plates from TV dinners that you've saved (you can also purchase them in your store) can be utilized very frequently to make excellent prepare-ahead meals. If, for instance, the family is having hamburger patties, cook enough of the hamburger ahead of time for at least two servings for the patient, blend with beef or beef and mushroom gravy, and place in two TV plates, adding blended potatoes and vegetable. Serve one that night—just heat in the oven while getting the meal for the rest of the family—and store the other one in the freezer for future use. However, after heating the frozen hamburger dinner, be sure to stir the meat portion, as the gravy has a tendency to settle on the top. This is not imperative; however, as mentioned under Helpful Hints in Chapter 1, attractive-looking meals are important, and the extra little effort to stir the meat mixture is well worth it in appearance and in tempting the appetite.

Homemade beef stew is something the whole family can eat, and it can be used for a semi-soft diet by cutting the stew meat, vegetables, and potatoes into very small cubes, approximately ½ inch square. The easiest way to cut the meat into such small pieces is to freeze the stew meat first, then, when partially thawed, and using a good sharp knife, it can readily be cut to that size. These ingredients can also be blended and are extra tasty as well as nourishing for a one-dish meal. Here again, extra portions may be placed in containers in the freezer for future use. Almost everyone has her own favorite recipe for beef stew, but for those who don't, there is one listed in Chapter 3, Semi-Soft and Blended Meals.

Meat loaf is another food the whole family can eat, as well as someone on a semi-soft diet, as long as gravy is added. For blending, just add beef gravy to the blender and a slice of meat loaf broken into bits for easy blending. Here again, extra portions may be frozen, either blended or made into a TV dinner for semi-soft or blended diet. There are several recipes for different types of meat loaf in the Semi-soft and Blended Meals chapter also.

Always remember, whenever possible, to freeze extra portions or meals for busy days, for variety, and for vacation use. Even canned soups can be blended and frozen for future use. Just be sure to mark containers showing contents of each, or you might have a few surprises when you defrost them!

As you become adjusted and accustomed to your new form of cooking, you will probably be able to adapt some of your family favorite meals so everyone will be happy, and you will also come up with some ideas of your own!

Just remember—don't feel housebound because of the problem in your family. For visiting, just take along one of those frozen meals you've already prepared (your hostess will be relieved of the problem of what to serve, and you'll all enjoy yourselves more). For vacationing, it is possible to rent one of the many housekeeping cottages with small kitchenettes, and they usually come equipped with the essential cooking utensils. If you are visiting family or friends for a few days or a week or so, you will be free to visit without unnecessary special cooking and blending.

So—get out your cooler—place however many pre-frozen meals your patient will require in it—and go!

# INDEX

Alcoholic beverages, 4–5, 104
Ale, 4–5
Apple-lime frost, 91
Apricot whip, 92
Asparagus with cheese sauce, eggs and, 8

Bacon
   eggs on rye (bread) with, 10
   -flavored liver, 19
Baked stuffed peppers, 36, 37
   with beef ravioli, 36
   with corned beef hash, 37
Baked stuffed tomatoes with celery cream sauce, 38
Banana cream pudding, Havana, 96
Bavarian cream pudding, orange, 97
Bean(s)
   green, casserole, meat and, 111–12
   lima, casserole, sausage and, 20
Beef
   corned, and vegetables, 109–10
   hash, corned
      baked stuffed peppers with, 37
      eggs and, 9
   Hungarian goulash, 18
   liver, bacon-flavored, 19
   meat loaf, 45–46
      with mushroom stuffing, 47–48
      top of stove, 56–57
   meat-za pie, 49–50
   pot pies, prepared frozen, 117
   ravioli, baked stuffed peppers with, 36
   and rice porcupines, 53
   roast, 43–44, 51–52
      chuck—skillet style, 43–44
      oven, 51–52
   steak, 74, 75, 76
      Italiano, 74
      with onion soup, 75
      with vegetable soup, 76
   stew, 41–43
   and zucchini, skillet, 54
   *See also* Meat(s)
Beer, 4–5
Beverages, 113

# INDEX

alcoholic, 4–5, 104
ale, 4–5
beer, 4–5
eggnogs, 104, 113
milk shakes, 104, 113
Blended meals, 39–88
  freezing and planning, 119–20
  *See also* Semi-soft and blended meals; specific foods, recipes
Boiled dinner with Daisy ham, old-fashioned, 64–65
Bountiful harvest spiced ham, 67
Bread pudding, 93
Broccoli
  with chicken cream sauce, 87
  in chicken divine, 78
Browning meat, 2–3
Butterscotch pudding, 98
  in whipped mocha mist, 98

Canned
  food, use of, 117–18
  fruits, 90, 92, 99, 100
  ham, oven-cooked, 66
  meats, 117
  soups, 3–4, 5, 40, 118
Carrots, 32, 109–10
Casserole(s)
  chicken and elbows, 25
  frank 'n' potato, 60
  meat and green bean, 111–12
  oyster-tuna, 32
  prepared, frozen, 116
  sausage and lima bean, 20
  tuna and elbow macaroni, 26–27
  Venetian, 70

Celery
  cream sauce, baked stuffed tomatoes with, 38
  -salmon loaf, 82–83
Cheese, 118
  deviled macaroni, 14–15
  and ham on rye, 63
  and macaroni with meat, 68
  pancakes, cottage, 13
  sauce, eggs and asparagus with, 8
  soufflé, 106–7
  veal Parmesan, 24
    economical, 21
Chicken, 3
  cream sauce, broccoli with, 87
  divine, 78
  and elbows casserole, 25
  legs, creamed, 79
  pot pies, frozen prepared, 117
Chiffon lemon dessert, 100
Chuck roast
  oven beef, 51–52
  —skillet style, 43–44
Corn and wiener roast, 58
Corned beef
  hash, 9, 37
    baked stuffed peppers with, 37
    eggs and, 9
  and vegetables, 109–10
Cottage cheese pancakes, 13
Creamed
  chicken legs, 80
  eggs, 108
    "quick," 12
  tuna fish and peas, 80

# INDEX

Cream of mushroom soup, ham slice with, 62
Cream pudding(s)
  Havana banana, 96
  orange Bavarian, 97
  peach cream dessert, 99
  tapioca, 94
Cream sauce
  celery, baked stuffed tomatoes with, 38
  chicken, broccoli with, 87
Creamy pork steak supper, 72
Creole hamburger on buns, 17
Curry (curried)
  lobster tails, tomato, 30
  tuna fish, 81
Custards, prepared, 89–90
    *See also* Desserts; Pudding(s)

Dairy products
  cheese soufflé, 106–7
  eggs. *See* Egg(s)
  for extra nutrition, 106–8
  macaroni, deviled, 14
  for semi-soft meals, 8–15, 106–8
  *See also* specific kinds, recipes
Daisy ham, old-fashioned boiled dinner with, 64–65
Desserts, 89–101
  apricot whip, 92
  bread pudding, 93
  cream tapioca, 94
  floating island deluxe, 95
  general information, 89–101
  Havana banana cream pudding, 96
  ice cream, 90, 113
  lemon chiffon, 100
  lime-apple frost, 91
  melon rings with strawberries, 101
  orange Bavarian cream pudding, 97
  peach cream, 99
  whipped mocha mist, 98
Deviled macaroni, 14–15

Economical veal Parmesan, 21
Egg(s), 3
  and asparagus with cheese sauce, 8
  and corned beef hash, 9
  creamed, 108
    "quick," 12
  poached in tomato sauce, 11
  on rye, 10
  terrapin, veal and, 23
Eggnogs, 104, 113
Eggplant Parmesan, 33–34
Equipment, 2, 39
Evaporated milk, 103–4, 108
  *See also* Milk; specific recipes

Fillets 'n' shrimp, 28
Fish. *See* Seafood (fish)
Floating island deluxe, 95
Frankfurter(s)
  corn and wiener roast, 58
  family style, 59
  'n' potato casserole, 60
  on rye, 16
  soup-kettle supper, 61
Frost, apple-lime, 91

# INDEX

Frozen foods, 90, 116–17, 119–22
  beef and chicken pot pies, 117
  beef stew, 120–21
  canned, 117–18
  casserole dishes, 116
  freezing and planning, 119–20
  meat loaf, 121
  soups, 116–17, 118
  vegetables, 116, 117–18
  See also specific recipes
Fruits (fruit desserts)
  apricot whip, 92
  canned and frozen, use of, 90, 92, 99, 100
  lemon chiffon dessert, 100
  lime-apple frost, 91
  melon rings with strawberries, 101
  orange Bavarian cream pudding, 97
  peach cream dessert, 99

Gelatin desserts
  apricot whip, 92
  lime-apple frost, 91
  orange Bavarian cream pudding, 97
  whipped mocha mist, 98
  See also Desserts; Pudding(s)
Goulash, Hungarian, 18
Gravy (gravies), use of, 3, 5, 40
Green bean casserole, meat and, 111–12

Haddock fillets 'n' shrimp, 28
Ham
  canned, oven-cooked, 66
  and cheese on rye, 63
  Daisy, old-fashioned boiled dinner with, 64–65
  and potatoes, scalloped, 69
  slice with cream of mushroom soup, 62
  spiced, bountiful harvest, 67
  See also Bacon; Pork
Hamburger(s)
  Creole, on buns, 17
  freezing and planning ahead, 120
Hash, corned beef
  baked stuffed peppers with, 37
  eggs and, 9
Havana banana cream pudding, 69
Hungarian goulash, 18

Ice cream, 90
  milk shakes, 113
Italiano steak, 74

Lamb dinner, one-dish, 71
Lemon chiffon dessert, 100
Lima bean(s)
  and sausage casserole, 20
  Venetian casserole, 70
Lime-apple frost, 91
Liver, bacon-flavored, 19
Lobster
  Newburg, 29
  tails, tomato curry, 30

Macaroni
  and cheese with meat, 68
  chicken and elbows casserole, 25
  deviled, 14–15

# INDEX

Hungarian goulash, 18
tuna and elbow casserole, 26–27
Meat(s)
　balls with noodles, tomato, 55
　for extra nutrition, 109–12
　and green bean casserole, 111–12
　loaf, 45–46
　　blending, freezing, and preparing ahead, 121
　　with mushroom stuffing, 47–48
　　top of stove, 56–57
　macaroni and cheese with, 68
　for semi-soft and blended meals, 41–78, 109–11
　　See also specific foods, recipes
　for semi-soft meals, 16–24
　　See also specific foods, recipes
　-za pie, 49–50
　See also Beef; Casserole(s); Chicken; Frankfurter(s); Ham; Lamb; Pork; Veal
Melon rings with strawberries, 101
Milk, 103–4, 106, 108
　eggnogs, 104, 113
　evaporated, use of, 103, 108
　extra nutrition, 103–4, 106, 108
　shakes, 104, 113
Mocha mist, whipped, 98
Mushroom
　pie, 35
　stuffing, meat loaf with, 47–48

Newburg
　lobster, 29
　sauce, shrimp 'n', 86
Noodles, tomato meat balls with, 55
　See also Macaroni
Nutrition, extra, 103–13

Old-fashioned boiled dinner with Daisy ham, 64–65
One-dish lamb dinner, 71
Onion soup, steak with, 74
Orange Bavarian cream pudding, 97
Oven beef roast, 51–52
Oven-cooked canned ham, 66
Oyster-tuna casserole, 31

Pancakes, cottage cheese, 13
Parmesan
　eggplant, 33–34
　veal, 24
　　economical, 21
Peach cream dessert, 99
Peas, creamed tuna fish and, 80
Peppers, green. See Baked stuffed peppers
Pie(s)
　beef and chicken pot, 117
　lemon chiffon dessert, 100
　meat-za, 49–50
　mushroom, 35
Poached eggs in tomato sauce, 11
Pork
　steak supper, creamy, 72
　and vegetable medley, 73
　See also Bacon; Ham
Potato(es)

'n' frank casserole, 60
scalloped, 88
ham and, 69
Pot pies, prepared frozen, use of, 117
Poultry. See Chicken
Prepared foods, use of, 115–18
Pudding(s)
bread, 93
cream tapioca, 94
Havana banana cream, 96
orange Bavarian cream, 97
packaged, use of, 89–90
peach cream dessert, 99
whipped mocha mist, 98
See also Gelatin desserts

"Quick" creamed eggs, 12
Quick seafood delight, 84

Ravioli, beef, baked stuffed peppers with, 36
Rice
and beef porcupines, 53
seafood delight, quick, 84
shrimp Creole, 85
Roast(s), 3
chuck—skillet style, 43–44
corn and wiener, 59
leftover, use of, 3, 23
oven beef, 51–52
veal, 77
Rye (bread)
eggs on, 10
frankfurters on, 16
ham and cheese on, 63

Salmon-celery loaf, 82–83

Sauce(s)
celery
cream, baked stuffed tomatoes with, 38
-salmon loaf, 82–83
cheese, eggs and asparagus with, 8
tomato, poached eggs in, 11
Sausage and lima bean casserole, 20
Savory veal steak, 22
Scalloped
ham and potatoes, 69
potatoes, 88
Seafood (fish), 26–31, 80–86
celery-salmon loaf, 82–83
delight, quick, 84
fillets 'n' shrimp, 28
lobster
Newburg, 29
tails, tomato curry, 30
for semi-soft and blended meals, 80–86
for semi-soft meals, 26–31
shrimp
Creole, 85
fillets 'n', 28
'n' Newburg sauce, 86
quick seafood delight, 84
tuna
curried, 81
and elbow macaroni casserole, 26–27
-oyster casserole, 32
and peas, creamed, 80
Semi-soft and blended meals, 38–88
dairy products, 106–8

# INDEX

desserts, 89–101
extra nutrition for, 106–13
general information, 1–5, 7, 39
meats and vegetables, 41–78, 87–88, 109–12
poultry, 78–79
seafood, 80–86
*See also* Semi-soft meals; specific recipes
Semi-soft meals, 7–38
dairy products, 8–15, 106–8
desserts, 89–101
extra nutrition for, 106–13
general information, 1–5, 7
meats and vegetables, 16–24, 32–38
poultry, 25
seafood, 26–31
*See also* Semi-soft and blended meals; specific recipes
Shrimp
Creole, 85
fillets 'n', 28
'n' Newburg sauce, 86
quick seafood delight, 84
Skillet
style chuck roast, 43–44
zucchini and beef, 54
Soufflé, cheese, 106–7
Soup(s), 3–4, 116–17
blending, 4, 118
canned and frozen, use of, 3–4, 5, 40, 116–17, 118, 121
-kettle supper, 61
mushroom
ham slice with cream of, 62
"quick" creamed eggs and, 12
onion, steak with, 75
vegetable, steak with, 76
Spiced ham, bountiful harvest, 67
Steak(s)
beef
Italiano, 74
with onion soup, 75
with vegetable soup, 76
chicken divine, 78
pork
creamy supper, 72
and vegetable medley, 73
veal
Parmesan, 24
economical, 21
savory, 22
Stew, beef, 41–43
freezing and preparing, 120–21
Strawberries, melon rings with, 101
Stuffed peppers, baked
with beef ravioli, 36
with corned beef hash, 37
Stuffed tomatoes with celery cream sauce, baked, 38

Tapioca pudding, cream, 94
Tomato(es)
curry lobster tails, 30
meat balls with noodles, 55
sauce, poached eggs in, 11
stuffed with celery cream sauce, baked, 38
Top of stove meat loaf, 56–57

# INDEX

Tuna
  curried, 81
  and elbow macaroni casserole, 26–27
  oyster casserole, 32
  and peas, creamed, 80
  TV dinners, use of, 116

Veal
  and eggs terrapin, 23
  Parmesan, economical, 21
  roast, 77
  steak, savory, 22
Vegetable(s), 32–38, 87–88
  blending, 32
  canned and frozen, 116, 117–18
  corned beef and, 109–10
  and meats, for extra nutrition, 109–12
  and pork medley, 73
  soup, steak with, 76
  *See also* specific kinds, recipes
Venetian casserole, 70

Welsh rarebit, canned, use of, 118
Whipped cream desserts, 89, 92, 97, 98
Wiener and corn roast, 58

Zucchini and beef, skillet, 54

4275